DEVELOPING COMMUNITY
NURSING PRACTICE

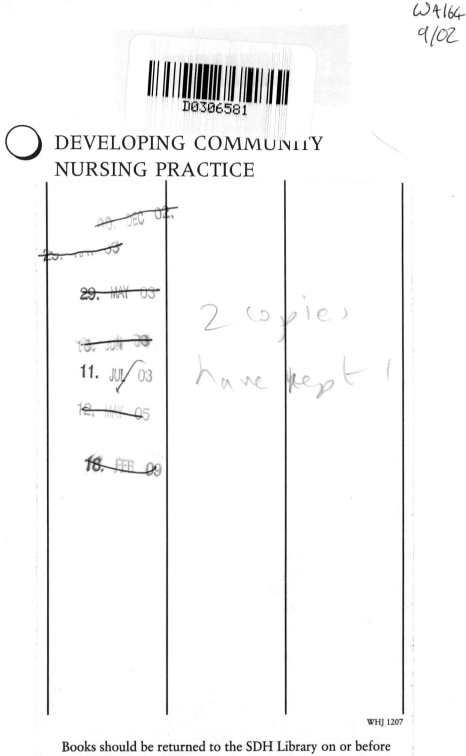

Books should be returned to the SDH Library on or before
the date stamped above unless a renewal has been arranged.

Salisbury District Hospital Library

Telephone: Salisbury (01722) 336262   extn. 4432 / 33
Out of hours answer machine in operation

DEVELOPING COMMUNITY NURSING PRACTICE

edited by
Sue Spencer, John Unsworth and
Wendy Burke

OPEN UNIVERSITY PRESS
Buckingham · Philadelphia

Open University Press
Celtic Court
22 Ballmoor
Buckingham
MK18 1XW

email: enquiries@openup.co.uk
world wide web: www.openup.co.uk

and
325 Chestnut Street
Philadelphia, PA 19106, USA

First Published 2001

A catalogue record of this book is available from the British Library

ISBN   0 335 20558 5 (hb)   0 335 20557 7 (pb)

Library of Congress Cataloging-in-Publication Data
Developing community nursing practice / edited by Sue Spencer, John Unsworth, and Wendy Burke.
       p.;   cm.
   Includes bibliographical references and index.
   ISBN 0-335-20558-5 (HB) – ISBN 0-335-20557-7 (PB)
   1. Community health nursing–Great Britain.   2. Community health nursing–Administration.   I. Spencer, Sue, 1961.   II. Unsworth, John, 1966. III. Burke, Wendy, 1964.
   [DNLM: 1. Community Health Nursing–organization & administration. 2. Nursing Care–organization & administration. WY 106 D489 2001]
   RT98 D49 2001
   610.73'43'0941–dc21   00-050178

Typeset by Graphicraft Limited, Hong Kong
Printed and bound in Great Britain by Biddles Ltd
www.biddles.co.uk

To our families

◯ Contents

List of tables and boxes

List of abbreviations

APEL	Accreditation for Prior Experiential Learning
AWBL	Accreditation of Work-Based Learning
CDT	Community Drug Team
CPT	community practice teacher
DRG	Drugs Reference Group
GP	general practitioner
HAZs	Health Action Zones
HIMPs	Health Improvement Programmes
INR	International Normalized Ratio
ITU	intensive therapy unit
NDUs	Nursing Development Units
NHS	National Health Service
NHS CRD	National Health Service Centre for Reviews and Dissemination
NP	nurse practitioner
PCT	Primary Care Trust
PDUs	Practice Development Units
PMS	Personal Medical Service
RCT	randomized controlled trial

Acknowledgements

The authors wish to extend their thanks to Eileen Morton for proofreading the various drafts of the text during its preparation and to Ray Pate (Risk Management Coordinator) Northumbria Healthcare NHS Trust for permission to reproduce the risk assessment tool in Chapter 4. Grateful thanks are also extended to the following people who contributed to the case studies in Chapters 6 and 7:

Nancye Carr, Practice Nurse, Birtley Community Nursing Team, Gateshead, UK;

Avril Haydock, Substance Misuse Services Manager, Bay Community NHS Trust, Lancaster, UK;

Robert Stanley, Senior Lecturer, Faculty of Healthcare Science, Kingston University and St. George's Hospital Medical School, London, UK.

Notes on contributors

Wilma W. Ayris – RGN, SCM, NDN, BA, MA Advanced Practice (Nursing), Clinical Lead Out of Hours Nursing Service, Northumbria Healthcare NHS Trust, North Tyneside, UK

Wilma Ayris is a district nursing sister with over 20 years' experience, much of this with the night nursing service in North Tyneside. She recently completed a Masters degree in Advanced Nursing Practice at the University of Northumbria, during which she developed a project to promote the use of advanced clinical assessment by district nurses out of hours, in order to provide a more responsive service to patients in the area.

Wendy Burke – MSc, BSc, RN, RHV, Service Development Manager, Whitley Bay Primary Care Group (Newcastle and North Tyneside Health Authority), UK

Wendy started her nursing career in 1982 in Dundee, Scotland. She has worked in the primary care setting for the last 12 years. A health visitor by background, she has held several clinical leadership posts, including clinical leader of an integrated community nursing team, and project manager for nurse prescribing at a regional level. Wendy has wide experience of practice development, notably in the areas of primary/ secondary care interface, integrated working and user perspectives. She has a particular interest in collaborative working as a way of dismantling the barriers between professional groups.

Professor Charlotte L. Clarke PhD, MSc, PGCE, BA, RN, Chair of Nursing Practice Development Research, University of Northumbria at Newcastle, Newcastle-upon-Tyne, UK

Charlotte Clarke has worked in nursing practice, education and research for almost 15 years. Most recently, she has managed a programme of research around the development of health and social care practice. This involves working very closely with care providers, using research and development activity to support learning about the needs and care of service users.

Glenda Cook – RGN, RNT, BSc (Psychology), MA (Medical Ethics), Senior Lecturer (Nursing Research), University of Northumbria at Newcastle, Newcastle-upon-Tyne, UK

Glenda Cook qualified as a registered nurse in 1982 and now works as a senior lecturer in nursing research. Her teaching and research activities are related to risk, law and ethics in professional health care practice, and the care of older people who are living in nursing homes.

Kate Henderson-Nichol – MA, RGN, RM, RHV, Adv. Dip Coun, Cert Health Ed. Independent Consultant, Primary Care, The Primary Care Consultancy, York, UK

Kate Henderson-Nichol has an extensive background in primary care. After becoming a lecturer/practitioner at York University, she went to the Queen's Nursing Institute as Professional Officer. Seconded to the Department of Health for three months, she later established her primary care consultancy. She continues to work nationally, supporting the development of innovative primary care practice.

Sue Spencer – MSc, BA, RGN, DN Certificate, PGCE, Senior Lecturer in Primary Health Care and Practice Development, University of Northumbria at Newcastle, Newcastle-upon-Tyne, UK

Sue Spencer has worked as both a district nurse and clinical nurse specialist before she took up her present post as senior lecturer. She has worked with a number of practitioners to support the development of practice and is currently seconded within the university to manage the clinical practice development accreditation scheme.

John Unsworth – MSc, BSc (Hons), BA, RGN, PGCE, Nurse Consultant – Intermediate Care, Northumbria Healthcare NHS Trust, Northumberland, UK

John Unsworth has worked in primary care for almost a decade. He has held several posts both in practice and education. A district nurse by background, John has extensive experience of practice development, and has worked with several community disciplines on practice and service development. His research interests include how organizations influence the development of clinical practice.

◐ Introduction

The latter part of the twentieth century saw a period of extensive and radical change in the structure and operating practices of the UK National Health Service (NHS). The dawn of the twenty-first century heralds a new era, during which the pace of change will be no less dynamic. The publication of the NHS Plan (Department of Health 2000a) presents new challenges for both NHS management and practitioners as the government seeks to modernize the delivery of health care. While the NHS Plan represents a top-down drive towards the development of clinical practice and patient-focused services, opportunities also exist for practitioners themselves to initiate change. The current climate of commissioning and quality provide a unique combination of challenges to nurses working within the community. On one hand, they can begin to visibly contribute opinions as to how services should be provided but on the other hand, they also have to demonstrate effectiveness, and develop their own practice and the way they deliver services. These two challenges may be seen by some as the straw that breaks the camel's back and sends them off into early retirement or long-term sick-leave. However, the contributors to this book have, collectively and differently, seen these challenges as the greatest opportunity community nurses have had to demonstrate their contribution to health benefits for the population.

The UK NHS is different, if not unique, in terms of its organizational structure. Not only is the health service the largest single employer in Europe, but it is also a highly complex bureaucracy, with many interconnecting constituent parts. Most organizations separate out the functions of manufacture and new product development/innovation. Rarely, if ever, is an employee on the shop floor expected to generate ideas about new ways of working, never mind plan their implementation and evaluate their effectiveness. Things are different within modern health care as health professionals are encouraged, and indeed expected, to develop clinical care and the services they provide. It could be argued that the NHS is a professional bureaucracy within a bureaucracy. Within a professional bureaucracy, workers are allowed considerable autonomy to apply their skills and knowledge to the needs of clients (Mintzberg 1979).

While it is widely accepted that nurses and other health care professionals are expected to develop their own practice, it is not until fairly recently that change management has become a key component of nurse education programmes. The practitioners themselves have faced particular challenges, not least because the NHS has rapidly moved away from tight management control of practice, leaving a void that practitioners were expected to fill. To what extent practitioners felt prepared to take on these challenges is debatable. Some staff were able to flourish in their new-found freedom to innovate, while others developed increasing frustration because of the lack of support available from increasingly distant line managers. Similarly those practitioners, who had in the past rested on their laurels, blaming the inability to develop their practice on their restrictive line manager, were now exposed and vulnerable.

Most practitioners who were either wishing to develop or who were forced to develop their practice turned to textbooks or articles for guidance on how to go about this process. While there are literally hundreds of texts on change and innovation, within the workplace, very few of these relate to health care or nursing practice. Most texts present change as a very linear process. As a result practitioners become disillusioned when their attempts to develop practice are thwarted or blocked. This book was born out of the frustration that, except for one or two texts, there is no acknowledgement of how highly complex the development of health care can become.

The text explores how community nurses can and do develop practice for the benefits of their patients/clients, and help those, feeling less confident, to grasp the nettle and put ideas into practice. We have aimed to dovetail theory and practice, to provide a basis for the development of practice, and throughout, the text vignettes and case studies are used to illustrate key concepts, by providing a snapshot of real life.

All of the examples, vignettes and stories in this book are drawn from real life developments in practice. However, most accounts have been fictionalized to allow for the illustration of key issues in practice development. The development of composite examples of this type is necessary in order that the negative aspects of practice development can be adequately portrayed. With the exception of two of the examples, where permission was granted for the use of people's real names, all names used within vignettes, stories and examples are pseudonyms.

The idea for this book came from a coffee room chat about the issues practitioners were wrestling with when attempting to respond to the need to develop existing practice. Practitioners and students alike were attempting to take practice forward, without visible frameworks with which to work. So what questions do practitioners ask about developing practice? They probably include the following:

- Where do I start?
- Who do I need to talk to before getting things started?
- What can go wrong, to whom and who's liable?
- Where do I access support and guidance?
- How do I sell my idea?

Answers to these practical questions should help the inexperienced or conscientious to take their first faltering steps in developing practice as well as prove a useful reference point for those already involved in practice development.

◯ Influences on nursing practice

Many might argue that the current climate of change and development in nursing practice is not new, and that nursing practice has always changed over time. However many of these changes, such as the nursing process and primary nursing, have been primarily top-down changes, and have been imposed on practitioners rather than organically derived from practitioner experience. Often these changes were not made in response to patient/client needs. Other changes, such as open visiting in hospitals, may appear to have been for the benefit of patients, but have often been developed without a full exploration of the impact on patient care or, indeed, on the visitors themselves.

In today's NHS any change in practice has to demonstrate both a clear rationale for implementation and a measurement of effectiveness. Therefore, changes cannot be made on a whim and, if they are, they are unlikely to be sustained, and certainly will not be taken up by others. All too often, in the past the sustainability of a development was sacrificed because of the desire for a quick fix or because of a need to be seen to do something about a problem, for example, developments that are initiated as a result of a complaint about patient care. In essence, developments in practice now need to be carefully thought through, and thoroughly planned. In Chapter 3, John Unsworth explores what you need to set in place to stand a sporting chance of successfully developing practice. Combined with meticulous planning, nurses are experiencing a shift in approach to developing health care services. Gone are the days when managers decreed what should be done and how, and this has been replaced with a patient-centred approach that encourages patient participation and user involvement (Department of Health 2000a). As there are fewer managers in today's health service, qualified nurses are expected to initiate developments in practice themselves. Thus the preparation for practice within higher education needs to equip practitioners with these skills.

◯ Nursing autonomy and the development of practice

Since the late 1980s a culture has begun to be developed within nursing, where instead of taking the lead from medicine, we have begun to take the initiative and respond to patient needs, without seeking permission from the medical hierarchy. Increased autonomy [within both nursing and practice development units] has demonstrated that nurses can work effectively to lead innovations in practice. Not only has this demonstrated that nurses can work autonomously, without detriment to patient experience but also those who have initiated these changes have disseminated their experience, so that we can all learn from their practice (see Pearson 1983 and Wright 1987). These early pioneers of nursing development felt very strongly that care, underpinned by nursing leadership, would improve patient care and the image of the nursing profession. These early innovations were soon adopted, and taken forward by the King's Fund, and over time 30 Nursing Development Units (NDUs) and Practice Development Units (PDUs) were established. It was envisioned that these NDUs and PDUs would be where the most innovative and creative nursing developments could happen, and were seen as 'test-beds' for developments (Gerrish and Ferguson 2000). These units could be seen as elitist, and other practitioners, outside the location of the units, might feel they have no role in the development of practice. This is exactly the issue we are addressing in this book. We, the editors, feel that all practitioners should be enabled to develop their ideas, and be given support and resources to be able to take ideas forward. They should not be constrained by organizational structure, and be allowed to take things forward only if they are a recognized development unit (be it nursing or practice led). Patient needs should be the focus of developments, and thus incorporated into service delivery, whether outside the boundaries of the four walls of a building or outside the boundaries of a defined team. Even development units might have their limitations. As Gerrish and Ferguson (2000) have stated, unless practice development is planned and integral to the strategic direction of the organization, it will be difficult to sustain. Developing elitist NDUs as the centres for development has not inculcated a culture of innovation and development. If individual practitioners are enabled and supported, it might be more likely to foster a climate within an organization that sees the development of practice not as the exception but as the typical activity of individuals and teams of professions. At last, many organizations are expecting nurses to take practice forward, and demonstrate the skills required to implement ideas, and subsequently evaluate them. Most job descriptions for qualified nursing posts now include the phrase 'ability to initiate and evaluate changes in practice'. This book is about supporting practitioners to do just that.

⃝ About this book

This book is divided into three parts. Part I looks at the things that may trigger a practitioner to develop practice. Part II examines the process of developing practice, and finally Part III addresses key issues that are common in many developments.

In the first chapter, John Unsworth explores the policy context of community nursing at the beginning of the twenty-first century. At a time of unprecedented change, both the structure of the Health Service and the prevailing philosophy underpinning care delivery are critically examined. The NHS is moving away from development that centred around the professionalization of certain occupations towards development that has a clear patient focus. With the devolution of responsibility for health care within the United Kingdom, we now have four health services, and this has been particularly challenging for the contributors to this book. We hope we have not been too Anglocentric, and we apologize if we have been. While the detail of management structures and policy may be different across the UK health departments, the paradigm shift within health care is universal. Patients and carers (rather than professional interests) have now been acknowledged as central to service development.

In Chapter 2 Charlotte Clarke and John Unsworth fully explore the various types of evidence that can be used to underpin the development of practice. The notion of evidence is explored, drawing upon a variety of sources (from traditional research approaches to the utilization of experience) as a basis for development. In writing the chapter, Charlotte and John have been careful not to be drawn into the debates about evidence-based practice, as this is more than adequately covered within other texts (see for example Hamer and Collinson 2000). Instead, the chapter forms a journey through the stages of practice development, mapping along the way the types of evidence a practitioner may need or draw upon at different stages.

In Chapter 3, John Unsworth explores the process of developing practice. He asserts that practice development is a specialized form of innovation, which has certain key attributes, including its strong patient focus. Several factors that may have a positive or negative impact on the development of practice are discussed, and the chapter provides practical guidance on how to turn an initial idea into a reality.

In Chapter 4, Glenda Cook and Wilma Ayris explore the very relevant issue of risk. The concept of risk has become familiar to many practitioners in an increasingly litigious society, and those pushing back the frontier within community nursing need to be fully aware of the risk implications of any developments. However, it's important to note that, with practice development, there is also a high level of risk related to inertia. Practitioners who fail to develop their practice may find themselves in a situation where they are placing patients, and themselves, at risk by continuing out-dated practices.

In Chapter 5, Sue Spencer explores the role education can and does play in the development of practice. The chapter debates, in an open and honest manner, whether education has a role, and if it has, then what should that role look like. By critiquing current approaches to nurse education, it is anticipated that this chapter should equip practitioners with the know-how to utilize education to develop practice while, at the same time, opening up the debate within education itself about the best approach.

Wendy Burke looks at various forms of power within Chapter 6. All nurses involved in practice development, will use or encounter power at some stage. Understanding the nature of this power is an important first stage in learning to manage the development of clinical care.

Finally, in Chapter 7 Kate Henderson-Nichol looks at new and different approaches to service delivery. Using in-depth case studies of developments in practice, coupled with analysis, Kate is able to articulate the issues around empowerment and collaborative working.

Chapters 6 and 7 cover all the eight specialist practitioner roles in community nursing, and in doing so, Wendy Burke and Kate Henderson-Nichol have sought to draw upon their own extensive experience to illuminate the issues critical to the development of nursing practice.

◯ How to use this book

We do not intend this book to be read from cover to cover (although you can if you wish) but readers are encouraged to dip in and out as required, to inform what you are currently involved with. Nor do we want you to concentrate on the topics covering your own specialist area of community nursing. We, the editors, have learnt so much from working with community nurses outside district nursing and health visiting and, as a result of our experiences, we urge you to do the same.

One of the criticisms that might be made about this book is that it portrays the development of practice in a neat, linear format. We appreciate that this is rarely, if ever, the case but writing a book round and round in circles, although an accurate metaphor for practice development, might not be an easy book to read! Developments in practice lead you down blind alleys and cul-de-sacs, and these are important factors to take into account. We do not discount these journeys, and hope they are represented in the vignettes we have used within this book. One of the best ways to learn about taking practice forward is to talk to others who have travelled the road before you, to see if there are any signs to adhere to, and if there are any hazards to avoid.

◯ A starting point

As with many new things in health care, the development of health care practice has yet to be fully integrated into the culture of most professions. However, many nurses are taking the lead, and as mentioned earlier, the development of more autonomy for nursing practice allows innovation to take place. What if you don't go with practice development? What does that mean, and can't I just carry on doing what I have always been doing? To answer that question let's look at an analysis of your options.

- *What if I ignore the whole idea and put my head in the sand?*
  In the past, this may have been a viable option. However, the pace of change in modern health care now dictates that all practitioners will be involved in some change or development at some time in their carers. It is also important to remember the risks associated with inertia, and that the failure to develop or to keep pace with new developments in practice could land a practitioner in deep water or, indeed, even in a court of law.
- *What about letting others get on with it?*
  This approach is fine, but don't be negative. At least support your innovative colleagues. In Chapter 3, John Unsworth identifies that those practitioners who get on with the day to day work, while others develop, are very valuable members of the team. Experience tells us that no one is totally against everything, even the most negative practitioner will be involved in a development which involves their favourite aspect of practice.
- *Let the students get on with it and leave me alone.*
  Education has a role to play in the development of practice, but practice should not be developed solely because of educational imperatives. As Sue Spencer states in Chapter 5, education and the

development of practice still have an ambiguous relationship and have much scope for development (Gerrish and Ferguson 2000).

We hope that we might have convinced sceptics that the development of practice is a good thing, and that ideas do not have to be big and ambitious. Often the simplest are the most effective, and if patient-led, they are the ones that will be noticed. If we are preaching to the converted, we trust you will dip in and out of this book, and that it proves a useful guide, and if you are a sceptic, we trust that you might dip your toe in the water and give practice development a try!

Sue Spencer
John Unsworth
Wendy Burke

Part (I) Triggering the development of practice

1) Developing primary care: the influence of society, policy and the professions

John Unsworth

◯ Chapter summary

The UK National Health Service, in common with most other public services, has undergone a period of considerable change and restructuring since the mid-1970s. It is fair to assume that these changes in policy and structure will continue in the future, as the NHS struggles to cope with rising demands and finite resources. At the same time, both the health professions and the practitioners themselves have had to become increasingly adept at coping with and meeting the challenges and opportunities presented by change. Within the NHS primary care was one area that saw the greatest stability through the 1970s and early 80s. Indeed many people perceived primary care as a sacred cow that should remain untouched. However, at the same time, people viewed primary care as a highly effective way of providing health care to large numbers of people at relatively low cost. All of this was to change when the Conservative government announced the most far reaching reforms ever to impact on the NHS (DoH 1989). These reforms were not only to change the way services were provided, but also were to reshape the way practitioners worked forever. These changes introduced a quasi-market with the creation of a purchaser–provider split, general practice fund holding and new self-governing hospital and community trusts. In many cases, practitioners were freed from the constraints of management and were encouraged, indeed expected, to develop practice. Some practitioners were well placed to meet these challenges and drive practice forward, while others were anxious and concerned about change. The latter response is understandable, when we consider that some community nurses experienced threats to their continued employment as general practice fundholders, exasperated by management, and sometimes even practitioner failings, took their business elsewhere. This chapter explores these and other contextual factors, which can either drive or suppress the development of practice. Any text that explores the current context of health care delivery, is likely to suffer as a result of policy change during the period between writing and subsequent publication. To minimize this, the chapter explores broad concepts, such as public health and social exclusion, which are illustrated by reference to current publications and policy. Throughout the chapter, policy as it relates to the four devolved National Health Services in the UK is explored. While some of this policy currently relates only to England, similar work is in progress in other countries to address similar issues and health problems.

◯ Context and its influence

There are numerous contextual influences on contemporary community nursing practice. The impact of such influences should not be under-estimated, because they not only help to shape the thought processes of practitioners, but they also create the climate for development. The nature of contextual factors, and their impact on the development of practice, can be summed up using the analogy of dropping a pebble into a rock pool. If there are calm weather conditions, the pebble will produce ripples within the rock pool which will dissipate out from the centre. However, if the sea is choppy, and there is a strong wind, the ripples will be either washed away, or will not be as effectively dissipated through the pool. A similar scenario can occur when developing practice. If the proposed development meets optimum conditions for its acceptance, and the development is in keeping with current policy, then it is more likely to be accepted and adopted by the organization and practitioners.

   The latter part of the twentieth century was characterized by a series of NHS reforms and changes in government policy. The majority of these had a significant impact on practice within primary health care, and many facilitated the development of practice. Taken together with changes within the nursing profession, and the changes in society, it quickly becomes clear that many community nurses have responded to the need to develop practice to meet the changing nature of health care delivery. While some practitioners have found it difficult to cope with the pace of change, it is evident that there is more change to come. With this is mind, it would seem that an awareness of the contextual influences on practice will enable the practitioner to be proactive in developing their clinical practice in line with both changing patient need and government policy.

◯ Professional changes

When considering professional contextual influences on the development of practice, it is worth examining the development of the various
branches of community nursing and how their roles have changed
over time. Some of the eight specialist practitioner branches are fairly
new, having been established as a result of various changes within the
National Health Service since its inception in 1945. Other branches
can trace their origins back much further to the nineteenth century.
Table 1.1 describes the origins of each of the eight branches of specialist
practice.

Early district nurses provided the majority of health care outside of
hospital, however, over a period of time this role has been eroded, with
the result that the traditional district nursing role centres on the provision of care to patients at home. Similarly, health visiting owes its
origins to the Victorian drive for sanitary reform, and this provides the
basis for the current role within public health. However, early health
visitors did not need to be nurses, and the need to lower the infant
mortality rate meant that health visitors concentrated their initial efforts
on mothers and children. Since the 1960s their role has evolved and has
moved from concentrating on under-5s to being more of a family visitor
although, for many, mothers and children have remained the central
focus.

Occupational health nursing has been shaped by legislation related to
health and safety, as well as both changes in employment practice, and
the move away from heavy industry into service industries and new
technologies. 'Traditionally, occupational health nurses were involved in
health and safety work and the treatment of illnesses and injuries' (Rossi
and Heikkinen 1990: 10). However, the role has evolved into preventat-
ive care to such an extent that they are now regarded as key public
health practitioners. Clearly the development of Health Action Zones,
with their emphasis on collaboration with business, will have a considerable impact on the role and function of occupational health nurses in
the next few years.

The growth of practice nursing owes its origin to changes within government policy and the increasing pressures on primary care. It could be
argued that the growth in the number of practice nurses was a direct
result of the failure of district nurses to extend their roles. This resulted
in district nurses feeling very threatened by the rapid expansion in the
number of practice nurses (Wood *et al.* 1994). While many practice
nurses confined their roles to the delivery of care within the general
practice, some have developed services that involve home visits and
assessment. Despite the concern about role erosion amongst district nurses,
in most cases practice nurses have carved themselves a distinct role in

Table 1.1 Origin of the eight branches of specialist community nursing practice

Branch of practice	First established	Initial role	Present role
Community Children's Nursing	1954 (While 1991)	Early services provided outreach services from acute care for children with chronic illness.	Community care of children with disabilities, special needs and chronic illnesses, as well as the identification of health needs amongst children in the community.
Community Learning Disabilities Nursing	mid-1970s (Sines 1995)	Supporting people with learning disabilities and their families who lived at home.	Care management for people living at home or resettled from institutions. Maximization of social inclusion and the promotion of health and independence.
Community Mental Health Nursing	1954	Aftercare for patients discharged from hospital, i.e. monitoring medications, supporting relatives etc.	Modern services provide specialist treatment outside of hospital, aftercare for those discharged from acute care, as well as specialist services, i.e. addictions.
District Nursing (nursing in the home)	Nurses cared for people in their own homes before 1834. Formally established 1887 – Queen's Nurses.	Early district nurses provided family care outside of hospital.	Shorter periods of hospital stay, rising number of elderly people and the trend toward caring for chronically ill people at home, has meant that district nurses spend more time caring for people at home.

General Practice Nursing	The first practice nurse was employed in 1913. However, it was not until the 1980s that the numbers of practice nurses increased.	Early practice nurses were involved in the administration of medicines and providing treatment room services.	In the past 10 years, practice nurses have developed considerable experience in chronic disease management, health education, screening and lifestyle change.
Health Visiting (Public Health Nursing)	1851	High infant mortality meant that early health visitors focused upon the care of mothers and children.	By 1956 the health visitor's role was extended into a family visitor.
Occupational Health Nursing	1872	Early occupational health nurses were concerned with accident prevention, the treatment of injuries and the screening of prospective employees.	Many occupational health nurses have been able to extend their role into disease and accident prevention.
School Nursing	1892	Early school nurses assisted medical staff with medical inspections, treatments and cleansing of school children.	School nurses have extended their roles in health promotion to address many of the new health problems that face young people.

chronic disease management and health promotion, which complements the services provided by other disciplines in primary care.

Until fairly recently, school nursing has followed developments within the School Medical Service. However, school nursing has broken free of the shackles which this association brought with it, and moved away from simple involvement in medical examinations, to take on a major public health role. This move is partly a response to the growth in the range and resourcing of primary care services, which has resulted in GPs taking more responsibility for child health surveillance (Department of Health 1996a). However, a major contribution has also been made by the realization that the health needs of school age children, have changed since the late 1980s. There is now a rising incidence of teenagers getting pregnant, being involved with drug abuse and having mental health problems, and action in relation to these problems now features prominently in the day to day work of the school nurse.

Community psychiatric nurses and learning disabilities nurses have developed since the late 1960s as a result of the policy of closing large institutions and moving towards more community based care. As a result, mental health practice has developed away from custodial care, toward the treatment and care of individuals within their own homes. Similarly, learning disability care has moved away from the provision of long term care to the maximization of independence and encouragement of self-care within a community setting.

Finally, community children's nursing is perhaps the newest of all of the community disciplines. Many practitioners in this field concentrate on the development of services that prevent admission to hospital or facilitate earlier discharge. Often this group of practitioners is involved with patients undergoing long term treatment or with chronic diseases.

Many of the community nursing disciplines have seen considerable development in their role and function over the last few years. However, some professionals have remained entrenched in the provision of services, which owes more to the historical origin of the professional group, than the health needs of today's population. The vignette in Box 1.1 illustrates this clearly in relation to district nursing involvement in the development of intermediate care services.

Box 1.1 illustrates how Alice resented having to provide care to patients in the new unit, because they should be the remit of the hospital service. Alice held the view that district nurses look after people in their own homes. What many community practitioners lose sight of, is that their roles are essentially the same, that they exist to assess health needs, and plan and deliver care to address those health needs.

Nursing staff working within primary health care have in the past been accused of being fiercely protective of their own work areas and roles. Mackenzie and Ross (1997) believe that the problems of professional

---

Box 1.1   District nursing involvement in intermediate care

In 1997 the government announced the availability of winter pressure money to relieve the pressure on acute beds over the winter months. One district nursing service had for a long time seen the need to establish beds that acted as a stepping stone between the general hospital and the community. This role and function had previously been fulfilled by the local community hospital, but over the last 20 years, many of these had been closed with the concentration of services on the general hospital site. The district nursing service, in partnership with the local authority, established a step-down unit in a local residential home. This unit was designed to take patients from acute wards and provide them with active rehabilitation prior to their discharge home.

   The unit proved to be very successful and continued well beyond the originally intended three months. While most of the district nurses in the area supported the unit and provided care to patients at weekends, some felt that the unit was yet another example of shifting services from secondary to primary care. Alice, one of the district nurses, opposed the establishment of such services because she felt that she had come into the community to look after people in their own homes and not to provide hospital care.

---

jealousy and unclear boundaries often mar the working relationships of practice nurses, district nurses and health visitors. This has often been referred to as tribalism, and occasionally results in fragmented care for patients who are often receiving interventions from a myriad of nurses, each sticking rigidly to their own individual roles. By the mid-1990s a new approach to overcoming some of the problems caused by tribalism were developed. This new approach centred on integrated working amongst nursing staff. The Community Practitioners and Health Visitors Association (CPHVA 1996: 2) defined integrated nursing as

   a team of community based nurses from different disciplines, working together within a primary care setting, pooling their skills, knowledge and ability, in order to provide the most effective care for
   their patients with a practice and the community it covers.

This new approach offered opportunities for primary care practitioners to develop services and practice outside of the constraints of traditional role boundaries. However, while the early exponents of integrated nursing had an opportunity to choose whether or not to be involved and own the process, the whole area of integrated nursing risks becoming a professional bandwagon that can be hijacked by other professional groups to manipulate the delivery of nursing services to their own ends. Nowhere is this clearer than in areas where integration has been used to replace practice nursing with an enlarged district nursing team. The whole philosophy of integrated nursing is the sharing of skills, knowledge and experience, and it should not involve the replacement of professional groups. Black and Hagel (1996) suggest that integration is not about people stepping directly into each other's roles, rather it was about increased flexibility and the prevention of overlap. It is important that staff involved in developing integrated teams are allowed to develop the team's philosophy and clearly define the parameters of integration. Additionally, the degree of integration should be measured in relation to the developments that occur within the team, rather than simply evaluating the process of integration.

Perhaps the most significant change agent in the development of clinical practice, was *The Scope of Professional Practice* (UKCC 1992a). This document set out principles which govern adjustments to practice and replaced the previous Chief Nursing Officer's guidance on the extended role of the nurse. Garbett (1996: 29) feels that by 'producing the scope document, the UKCC has contributed to a less restrictive atmosphere in which nurses have taken on more complex roles'. The principles outlined by *The Scope of Professional Practice* require the nurse to ensure that practice is directed towards meeting patient's needs. Therefore any development in practice must have a clear patient focus, and not simply be about the delegation of a task from one professional group to the other. The holistic imperative, which is a central tenet of *The Scope of Professional Practice*, went some way towards overcoming the tensions between the development of practice and concerns about the medicalization of nursing (Edwards 1995). Under *The Scope of Professional Practice*, the practitioner is required to develop and maintain the skills and competence to meet the patients' needs, acknowledge limitations in skill and competence, and ensure that enlargement or adjustment in role does not compromise existing practice (UKCC 1992a). A review of the implications of *The Scope of Professional Practice* (UKCC 2000) identifies the need to strengthen support mechanisms for practitioners who intend to develop their role. Clearly practitioners need support to develop protocols and guidelines, which are designed to manage and minimize risk, as well as support aimed at monitoring performance through regular clinical supervision.

Within community practice, *The Scope of Professional Practice* had less of an impact than it did within secondary care, mainly because the development of practice, within this context, was driven by the 'new deal for junior doctors' (NHS Management Executive 1991). However the medical profession is still having an influence on the development of community practitioner's roles. The continual drop in the number of doctors entering GP training, and the problematic nature of recruiting GPs to work in inner city or remote areas, has served as the impetus for the development of the nurse practitioner (NP) role. The development of such roles has increased in the late 1990s, with the advent of nurse-led Personal Medical Service (PMS) pilots and walk-in centres. The concept of a NP role is not new and the concept first originated in the USA in the 1960s, in response to a shortage of primary care physicians. Pearson *et al.* (1995: 157) describe how

'doctors and managers here, like their colleagues in America before them, have begun to wonder if some more flexible community nurses might be able to cost effectively take on some of the roles they are unable to fulfil adequately'.

Drury *et al.* (1988) describe how nurse practitioners carry out their work safely and effectively. The care provided is often holistic in nature with assessment, diagnosis and treatment being combined with health promotion and advice. Nurse practitioner roles in primary care have developed in several areas, including minor ailments and chronic disease management. One of the main obstacles to such posts reaching the full potential has been the inability to prescribe. This has resulted in some practitioners developing imaginative, and occasionally illegal, methods of obtaining medications for patients. However, in March 2000 the Department of Health (DoH 2000b) announced plans to expand the groups of independent prescribers, and create a new category of dependent prescribers, thus allowing nurses a greater role in chronic disease management.

As part of the government's drive to create more accessible primary care services, the Department of Health announced the creation of 20 pilot walk-in centres. These centres would provide members of the public with the opportunity to see a doctor or nurse between the hours of 7 a.m. and 10 p.m., often without an appointment. Services provided would include advice and treatment for minor conditions. Walk-in centres are obviously well placed to meet the health needs of specific parts of the population, who find normal general practice opening hours restrictive. The government made it clear that such services are designed to complement rather than replace existing provision. Despite these reassurances, the British Medical Association (BMA 1999) raised concerns about the establishment of additional services when the provision of general practice services were already underfinanced. The BMA stated that the UK has the lowest number of doctors per head of the population in Europe, and this was the fundamental problem. The BMA called for more GPs to cope with increasing demands, rather than the establishment of complementary services.

Similarly, Personal Medical Service (PMS) pilots offer new opportunities for nurses by altering the power balance between the professions. Some of the first PMS pilots are nurse-led, and employ salaried GPs. These are especially useful in inner-city areas, or for services providing health care to disadvantaged groups, such as homeless people. PMS pilots, and the opportunities they present for nursing are discussed later in this chapter.

◯ Policy changes

Since the early 1980s, there have been major changes in health policy which have shaped the development of both the NHS and the clinical practice within it. Most of the policy changes can be grouped together into the following broad categories:

- changes in the structure, role and function of the NHS or NHS bodies;
- public health strategy and strategies designed to promote social inclusion;
- policy and strategy focused on service development or professional groups.

As well as the specific government policy documents, several other areas have had an impact on community nursing practice. These include the rise in the number of patients undergoing day surgery, as well as the range of procedures that are now performed using such surgery. In 1991 37.7 per cent of all general and acute patients underwent day surgery. This number rose to 56.2 per cent by 1996 (NHS Executive 1996a). Many of these patients are followed up by district nurses at home, for wound checks and dressing, pain control and post-operative advice. Similarly, the government's waiting list initiative has resulted in a drive for faster patient discharge to allow greater numbers of patients to undergo surgery. Both of these changes come at a time when there are fewer acute beds than ever before. Some of these beds have been lost because of changes in technology, treatments, or the way in which surgery is performed. In 1980 there were 140,000 acute beds in the NHS. This had fallen to 110,000 by 1998. In total, more than 100,000 beds have been lost since the 1960s (DoH 2000c). In 1996 the Chief Nursing Officers of the UK Health Departments met to discuss a vision for nursing and midwifery into the twenty-first century. The resulting consultation document, The Heathrow Debate (DoH 1996b) sets out the skills and knowledge which nurses will need into the new millennium. At the time, they predicted that by 2002 some 60 per cent of surgery would be done on a day case basis. As a result, the pressures this brings to the community nursing service are likely to grow, and the number of acute beds is likely to fall still further.

The reduction in acute beds has also provided several opportunities for many community practitioners. The establishment of intermediate care services in many parts of the UK is a direct result of the need to facilitate the best use of acute beds, as well as provide structured rehabilitation to elderly people prior to discharge home. Steiner and Vaughan (1996: 29) describe how

> intermediate care is seen as a specific service, aimed at meeting the needs of those people, who are physiologically stable, but could improve the quality of their lives, increase their ability to live independently and minimise their longer term dependence on health care services through timely, intensive therapeutic input.

The term 'intermediate care' has been used to describe a number of methods of service delivery, including hospital at home, facilitated discharge and step-up units. Central to all forms of intermediate care is the concept of transition between care and home and restoration of health or independence (Steiner and Vaughan 1996). District nurses in particular have been quick to become involved in such initiatives by either coordinating the service, or playing a role as part of the multidisciplinary rehabilitation team. The Audit Commission report on district nursing (Audit Commission 1999a: 24) suggests that 'district nurses can respond to unmet needs in innovative ways and relieve the pressure on acute services, when additional resources are made available'. The National Beds Inquiry (DoH 2000c) suggests an expansion of intermediate care services. If the government does expand such services, district nurses could find themselves at the forefront of the development of services, such as hospital at-home schemes, facilitated discharge and rapid response.

Of all of the changes to the NHS that have taken place in the late twentieth century, perhaps the most significant was the 1990 NHS and Community Care Act. This paved the way for the establishment of NHS Trusts and the purchaser/provider split. The same Act also set the scene for the creation of new community care arrangements, the impact of which will be discussed later in this chapter. The creation of this internal health market, perhaps more than any other contextual influence, had the greatest impact on the development of nursing practice. Hospital and community services were forced to compete with each other for contracts from both health authorities and a new group of purchasers, general practice fundholders. The development of competition between NHS organizations has been heavily criticized by many authors (Ranade 1997) but this development also prompted both managers and practitioners to examine the services they provide, and make alterations to them, so that they would be more attractive to potential purchasers. The result of this was that practitioners were often freed from the constraints placed on practice by their manager, and services often became much more responsive as a result. Ranade (1997) describes how GP fundholders were effective in securing improvements in the quality of services provided to their patients.

However, the development of competition also resulted in several major problems. NHS organizations became increasingly secretive about their planned developments, and often were reluctant to share their experiences with others. As a result, duplication of services occurred and a considerable amount of time and energy was wasted reinventing the wheel. During this period of change, community nurses were particularly concerned about the changes which GP fund holding brought. Often GP fundholders used their newfound power, in terms of purchasing, to develop new services and ways of working. In some areas, these were welcomed by practitioners, while in others, the practitioners were constantly under a cloud because of the ever present threat that the GP fundholder could take their contract for nursing services elsewhere. During this period, there were several high profile contract losses, which often did not result in a change of staff for the practice, but meant that the staff were employed by a different NHS Trust. These moves of contract were not without their problems, principally because of the logistical arrangements for the provision of support services, such as loan equipment, continence supplies and out of hours cover.

More recently, the White Papers produced by the UK Health Departments (DoH 1997a; Scottish Office 1997; Welsh Office 1998a; Northern Ireland Office 1998) have advocated a move away from GP fund holding to the development of locality commissioning bodies. These bodies (Primary Care Groups in England and Northern Ireland, Local Health Groups in Wales and Local Health Care Co-operatives in Scotland) are formed from groups of Primary Health Care Teams, serving a population of between 25,000 and 150,000 people. Most of these bodies cover natural communities, and Local Health Groups in Wales are formed around unitary local authorities. The purpose of the groups are to:

- assist in the planning of a programme to improve the health of the local population;
- actively promote the health of the local population;
- commission new health and, in some cases, social services for their local population;
- monitor performance of local health services;
- develop primary care by joint working across practices;
- better integrate primary and community health services, as well as working closely with other health and social care providers.

In England, the groups can exist at several different levels, either as part of the Health Authority, as independent bodies accountable to the Health Authority or as independent Primary Care Trusts. In Scotland Local Health Care Co-operatives (LHCCs) are bodies within newly formed Primary Health Care Trusts. These trusts were brought about by the merger of existing community services provided by NHS Trusts and LHCCs, although GPs continue as independent contractors.

Local health commissioning is not new, and the new arrangements are built on previous total commissioning and multifund pilots. The new arrangements have allowed new players to be brought into the commissioning process. The boards of the new commissioning groups and cooperatives are made up of GP, nurse, local authority social services and lay representation. For many nurses, involvement in commissioning is a new experience, although some people, notably Willis (1998) have concerns that nurses do not have the same supporting infrastructure or experience of the process of commissioning as their GP colleagues. The appointment of nurse representatives has been handled in a number of different ways; some have been elected by their peers, while others have been appointed by the members of the board (usually general practitioners). This process has resulted in considerable debate, and it is unclear whether in every case the people with the right skills, knowledge and experience have been appointed. There has also been considerable debate about whether every professional discipline is fully represented, and this has opened up old divisions within the profession. It is not uncommon to find that the board member is a district nurse or health visitor, and groups such as practice nurses and midwives find that they are not represented. However, the important thing about being in such a group is that the person is there to represent the needs of the local population during the formulation of the health improvement programme, and not necessarily the professional group to which they are aligned.

Further concerns have been voiced about the move towards Primary Care Trust status in England. Many community nurses are worried that this will mean they will be employed directly by GPs. The truth is that, were a Primary Care Group to become a Primary Care Trust, staff would be employed by a NHS Trust in the same way as they are currently. The staff would transfer to this new trust on their present contract of employment with the same terms and conditions (Young 2000). Primary Care Trusts are likely to be very different beasts to their PCG forerunners. Whereas in many PCGs, general practitioners hold the balance of power, a PCT would be made up of a Trust Board of executive and non-executive directors. The chairperson of these new trusts would be appointed by the relevant health department, and would be accountable to them. Below the Trust Board, a PCT Executive would be established. This group would be similar to the composition of the PCG, and it is likely that the executive would be responsible for commissioning services. Essentially, staff have very little to fear from PCT status, and indeed, it could signal an end to many of the artificial divisions which have caused so many problems in the past, although there is still no provision for automatic transfer of practice nurses from practice to trust employment. Imagine having just one body responsible for primary care services across a locality with all staff working towards the health improvement programme developed by that trust, the local community and the health authority. Such a move has the potential to facilitate the development of integrated services and fully integrated teams.

Another new area is the development of Personal Medical Service (PMS) pilots. These pilot projects are intended to give health authorities and providers, particularly GPs, nurses and NHS Community Trusts, different options for addressing primary care needs. The Department of Health in England (DoH 1998a) describes how such pilots should be used to provide faster, more convenient and more widely accessible primary care services. PMS pilots provide an alternative to the national GP contract as a means of contracting for the provision of general medical services. Two types of pilot exist: PMS pilot status involves the provision of those services patients would normally expect from their GP, while PMS plus includes those services, as well as the services sometimes provided by hospital or community health services. Primary Healthcare Development (1999), a primary care management consultancy company, describes how PMS pilots are more flexible, and are particularly suitable for anyone wishing to better target particular client groups, expand the range of primary care services, or wishing to provide more flexible employment options for GPs.

The first wave of pilots commenced in April 1998 with a further wave in 1999. The government particularly encouraged bids from community nurses or NHS Trusts. The first wave of pilots involved a number of innovative services, including nurse-led sites where the nurses employed salaried general practitioners to assist in the delivery of services. Other pilots targeted often neglected sections of society including the homeless and travelling populations. PMS and PMS plus pilots present a number of opportunities and threats for nursing staff. Many sites have encouraged active nurse involvement, both in needs assessment, and service delivery, and this has, without doubt, improved the delivery of integrated care. Additionally, these pilots have improved the provision of services to socially excluded groups and in areas of deprivation, where it is often difficult to recruit GPs. However, some former GP fundholders have seen PMS status as a way of regaining some of the freedoms they have lost since the demise of fundholding. PMS plus pilots also carry potential threats to the nurses' employment prospects, as the practice has several options of how to integrate community health services into the pilot. PMS plus sites can either employ nursing staff directly, or second staff from community trusts.

The NHS Plan published by the government in August 2000 (DoH 2000a), provides further impetus for reform with historic sustained increases in funding, and a vision of a health service for the twenty-first century designed around the patient. 'The vision of this NHS Plan is to offer people fast and convenient care delivered to a consistently high standard. Services will be available when people require them, tailored to their individual needs' (DoH 2000a: 17). Developing the skills and potential of staff is a fundamental part of the plan and it offers huge opportunities for community nurses to develop new ways of working, so that modern patient-centred services become a reality.

◯ Promoting public health and social inclusion

Each of the countries which make up the UK have produced a blueprint for public health (Northern Ireland Office 1997; Welsh Office 1998b; DoH 1999a; Scottish Office 1999). These documents set out an ambitious programme to improve the health of everyone, with a particular focus upon improving the health of the most disadvantaged in society. All of the documents recognize the link between ill health and socioeconomic factors, and as a result, the public health strategies are tied up in other government initiatives, that is, the New Deal. The English White Paper *Saving Lives: Our Healthier Nation* (DoH 1999a) suggests that the government is tackling inequality with a range of initiatives on education, welfare to work, housing, transport and the environment.

All of the public health strategies share several cornerstones, including social inclusion, collaborative working, better information to facilitate and encourage individual responsibility, and sustainability of action and health gains. Social inclusion is a key factor in several government policies. In 1997, the Prime Minister announced the establishment of a social inclusion unit as part of the Cabinet Office. The purpose of this unit is to help improve government action to reduce social exclusion, by producing 'joined-up' solutions to 'joined-up' problems. Essentially, the unit works on cross-departmental problems that have a bearing on social exclusion, for example, teenage parents, poor neighbourhoods etc. Scotland, Wales and Northern Ireland all have similar work in progress to tackle social exclusion within their own countries. Each of the public health strategies sets specific targets; most of these centre around reducing deaths from cancer, heart disease, accidents and addressing mental health problems. The National Assembly for Wales set a total of 15 targets for the next five years, including reducing low birth weights, smoking and dental caries. The Welsh strategy acknowledges that they are starting from a lower baseline in relation to health than the rest of the UK, stating that health in Wales is worse than in most parts of the UK. The strategies suggest a number of ways in which health could be improved, including the development of healthy citizen programmes to assist people to help themselves and manage their own illnesses. These initiatives also include the development of NHS Direct, Healthy Living Centres funded via the National Lottery, and the creation of Health Action Zones within England.

The improvement of existing services to ensure there is equity of provision would be tackled in several ways. First, the development of National Service Frameworks will assist health commissioners to match service provision to national standards. At a local level, services will be improved through the development of Health Improvement Programmes (HImPs). These programmes will be developed jointly by local commissioning groups, health authorities and local authorities. HImPs will be effective vehicles for major and sustained impact on health problems in every locality. As well as looking at the overall health of the local population, they will focus action upon people who are socially excluded and need the most support.

In 1997 the government announced the creation of a number of Health Action Zones (HAZ) within England. Similar initiatives are also in progress in Northern Ireland. The purpose of these zones was to bring together all those organizations who contribute to the health of a local population and get them to collaborate on the development and implementation of a locally agreed strategy for improving the health of local people.

Eleven Health Action Zones were created on 1 April 1998. The key objectives of each of the HAZs are to reduce health inequalities, improve services and build sustainable capacity from local resources. HAZ status exists for between five and seven years, and the zones are expected to put programmes in place to deliver improved health in some of the most deprived communities through collaborative working. The government believe that the tackling of health inequalities is a key element of creating social inclusion (DoH 1997b). All of the Health Action Zones address three broad strategic objectives. These are to identify and address the public health needs of the local areas through the empowerment of people, building on the communities' strengths and focusing upon those whose needs are greatest. The zones should also work towards increasing the effectiveness, efficiency and responsiveness of local services, and developing partnerships for improving people's health.

All four of the public health strategies recognize the important public health role of community nursing staff. There is a recognition that the public health role of the health visitor, school nurse and occupational health nurses needs to be strengthened if the targets are to be met. Health visitors will have a key role in supporting families through programmes such as Sure Start. Sure Start is a cross-government strategy for children under 4 and their families in areas of disadvantage. The aim of the programme is to improve opportunities for children by providing better access to childcare, health, early years education and parenting support. The programme is built upon the idea of partnership between health, social services and the local community, and the guidance is very clear that Sure Start programmes must complement existing services. The Department of Health (DoH 1999b) outlines how the government is determined that Sure Start should set new standards of interagency and interdepartmental working, breaking down barriers that prevent families receiving the comprehensive and coordinated services they need. Health visitors play a major role in achieving the objectives of the Sure Start programme. In particular, they are concerned with improving the social and emotional development of children through support for parents, the promotion of bonding between the parents and the child, the early identification of health and behavioural problems, and the promotion of play and language development. Sure Start trailblazer areas were established in 1999, and over the next three years there will be 250 projects established with funding of £452 million. The projects have very clear targets to be met during their lifetime. These include reductions in the number of 'at-risk' registrations on the child protection register, low birthweight babies and children admitted to hospital with illnesses or injuries. Additionally, targets have been set to increase the number of children with normal speech and language development, and that all children will have access to quality play and learning activities.

The government has announced an ambitious programme to tackle some of the causes of social exclusion (Social Exclusion Unit 1998). The approaches identified are not without their problems, as they can create artificial boundaries within communities and further compound social isolation. The initial focus of the Social Exclusion Unit was to develop policy to reduce truancy and school exclusion, rough sleeping, teenage pregnancy and stimulate neighbourhood renewal. A range of cross-departmental initiatives were introduced, such as the new deal for communities programme with resources of £800 million to support redevelopment. The money was provided to encourage business, reduce unemployment, reduce crime and provide better housing.

The government's drive to regenerate the poorest communities (Social Exclusion Unit 1998) can lead to the development of animosity between the perceived 'winners' and 'losers'. Approaches such as the Single Regeneration Budget (SRB) and the associated competition to win funding does little to overcome such feelings (Hopkins *et al.* 1997). The challenge for the agencies involved is how these negative reactions can be avoided. Anecdotal evidence from some of the Sure Start trailblazer areas suggests that many of the existing health visitors are envious of their Sure Start colleagues, who are getting additional resources, study leave and smaller caseloads.

Another major aspect of the public health strategy in England is the Healthy Schools programme. This is a cross-government initiative between the Department of Health and the Department for Education and Employment (DfEE). The DfEE defines a healthy school as one that is successful in helping pupils to do their best, and build upon their achievements (DfEE 1997). The initial part of the programme involved the establishment of eight education and health partnerships where schools, parents, local education authorities and health authorities join forces to drive up standards of health. A key part of the programme was the establishment of a Healthy School standard. This standard is adaptable enough to reflect local needs and best practice, and involves staff, young people, statutory and non-statutory agencies and community groups in the planning, development and evaluation of activities. It is anticipated that all local education authorities will be involved in an accredited education and health partnership by 2002. In addition to the standard, another major feature of the Healthy Schools programme is work to improve the health of teachers. The initial work in this area was to involve teachers in the identification of health needs and plan development to meet these needs. This involved six consultative conferences during 1999. The main findings of this consultation was the need to improve occupational health provision for teachers, with attachment of services to local schools, the need to involve staff, to improve their health and their working environments, and better coordination of organizational change.

In 1998 the Ministerial Group on the Family produced a consultation document *Supporting Families* (Home Office 1998a) which set out the government's approach to supporting families in England, Wales and Northern Ireland. The document centres on five areas where the government feels it can make a difference. These include the provision of advice and support, improving family prosperity, improving the balance between work and home, strengthening marriage and tackling some of the serious problems of family life, for example domestic violence and school age pregnancy. The document suggests that health visitors have a key part to play in supporting families, and that their role should be extended beyond health in its narrowest sense, to supporting families more generally. While the document acknowledges that the scope of health visiting practice could be expanded to include toddler training groups, school settling groups and work with teenagers, there is also acknowledgement of the pressure on existing services, and the need for additional funding and an expansion in the number of health visitors. The initial consultation document failed to acknowledge the important contribution school nurses could also make to the development of support for families, and the tackling of teenage pregnancy. However, the subsequent consultation (Home Office 1999) highlighted the way in which this professional group could assist in the support of families.

○ The impact of policy and strategy on individual professional groups

There have been numerous reports and consultation documents, which have and will continue to influence the development of practice within professional groups. Some of these documents have been discussed earlier in this chapter, while others, related to school nursing, occupational health, mental health and community children's nursing practice, will be discussed later. One group of reports, which will impact on all community nursing disciplines, are the nursing strategies produced by the English, Welsh and Northern Ireland Health Departments (Department of Health and Social Services 1999; DoH 1999c; National Assembly for Wales 1999). These reports recognize the rapidly changing context of care delivery, and aim to equip nursing staff with the skills and knowledge to develop and innovate in areas of practice. The reports acknowledge the urgent need to provide both short and long term solutions to the current recruitment difficulties faced by nursing. They suggest new pay structures, increased student nurse training places and encouraging more nurses to return to practice. All of these strategies suggest strengthening both pre and post-registration nurse education, and the development of a modern career structure. This includes the development of new nurse consultant posts, which are designed to allow highly experienced practitioners to stay in clinical practice. The development of these posts, within primary and secondary care, should strengthen the leadership, research, education and promote the development of clinical practice. Hesketh (1999) suggests that the ever-changing structures in the community may result in problems in deciding the greatest areas of need, in relation to the introduction of these posts. However, there are several possible opportunities to promote the development of key areas of professional practice. For example, a nurse consultant post in school nursing or health visiting could assist in the development of the public health role of practitioners.

As a professional group, school nursing has seen the erosion of many of its traditional activities, such as medical checks, as many of these activities are now undertaken by general practitioners. The Department of Health (1996a) in their report *Child Health in the Community: A Guide to Good Practice* identified that school health services should now be more selective, concentrating on health advice, the identification of special educational needs and health promotion. In some areas these changes and the subsequent guidance has resulted in cutbacks in the provision of school nursing. This has occurred despite the fact that school nurses have been quick to grasp the opportunities extended to them in developing the public health side of their role. In 1995 the Chief Nursing Officer for England initiated three separate research projects to look at aspects of the school nurse's role. A summary of these projects, and recommendations for the future provision of school nursing, were made in a report published by the Department of Health and the Queen's Nursing Institute (Bagnall and Dilloway 1997). The report highlighted areas of good practice in relation to school health profiling and health questionnaire interviews. It was suggested that the information from these two processes could assist in the commissioning process by allowing for the better targeting of resources. The information gleaned from profiling and interviews could also be used to formulate outcomes, thus allowing school nurses to better evaluate the outcomes of their interventions. The report also suggested that better skill mix within school nursing could free up time for more health promotion and public health activity. However, while many of the examples of good practice seemed to have been widely implemented across the country, skill mix remains a thorny issue for many school nursing services.

More recently, the Community Practitioners and Health Visitors Association (CPHVA 2000) have collaborated with several nursing organizations to develop a national framework for school nursing. The purpose of the framework was to clarify the range and scope of school nursing services and focus upon how school nursing could move forward. The review team believed that 'achieving improvement in children's health demands that we go beyond the boundaries of conventional health services' (CPHVA 2000: 5). The report suggests that the health needs of school-age children can be divided into four broad categories. These are healthy lifestyles, mental health, children with chronic or complex health needs and vulnerable children. However, the provision of services is affected by problems with the current workforce, for example inflexible working, little skill mix and leadership. Finally, the report suggests that the core programme of child health surveillance should be re-examined and flexible working should be encouraged through improved training for staff and the introduction of skill mix.

Nursing practice in the field of learning disabilities has been heavily influenced by the continuing resettlement of people from long-stay hospitals back into the community. The Department of Health (1999d: 8) outlines how the 'continuing movement away from long-term care in hospital, to alternative forms of care, had been guided by policy established long before the reforms and specialist guidance of the early 1990's'. The drive towards community care for people with learning disabilities has presented several problems for community learning disabilities nurses; amongst these problems are working with multiple agencies such as the private sector and local authorities. However, many practitioners have made good progress with joint working, and integrated health and social care teams are now commonplace. Indeed, the Department of Health discussion document *Partnership in Action* (DoH 1998b) puts forward proposals for closer working between health and social care; many of the examples given in this document are from learning disabilities teams.

In 1999 the Department of Health (DoH 1999d) undertook a study to assess progress towards the models of social care and health service envisaged in government policies of the 90s. The report identified that agencies subscribed to the principles of social inclusion, citizenship and community living. However difficulties were identified in relation to the provision of care for people with complex needs. They also found that 60 per cent of users living with carers did not have respite care, and that congregate care in group homes still predominates over and above all other forms of community living. Other problems involved access to mainstream health care for people with learning disabilities, and the need to formalize policies to protect users from abuse.

In occupational health nursing, the publication of a discussion document related to the development of a 10-year Occupational Health Strategy for Great Britain (Health and Safety Executive 1998) is likely to have far reaching effects on the role and function of occupational health nurses in the future. The discussion document outlines how, despite progress in eliminating previously common occupational illnesses, there is the need to take account of demographic and employment changes, that is, smaller firms, an older workforce, and greater public expectations. The HSE recognizes that people are still made ill by their work, yet they acknowledge that occupational ill health is preventable. The discussion document attempts to identify why people are still made ill by work activities, and suggests that some of this can be attributed to a lack of accountability for risk assessment and reduction. This is further compounded by the provision of poor quality advice to employers and employees, and little central information about the risks which the workplace can pose. The document goes on to suggest seven strategic aims which contain detailed targets for both the HSE and other interested parties. The aims include the introduction of sustainable procedures, systems and campaigns to address specific occupational health issues and the assessment of workplace health and potential risks to the health of employees.

Clearly, these aims have major implications for occupational health nurses. These practitioners are ideally placed to assess the general health of the workforce, identifying specific health needs and unmet health needs. This information can be used as a basis for the development of a health improvement plan, around which sustainable interventions and campaigns can be organized, delivered and evaluated. Additionally, risk identification and management is already a key part of the occupational health nurse's role. The ENB (1998: 14) describes how

occupational health nurses can work with the employer to identify, eliminate or control risks to health of employees, by undertaking targeted risk assessments to explore the probability of risk outcomes, including injury or disease.

Other strategic aims in the discussion document include the collection of occupational health information, and the training and education of employers/employees. Both of these aims already form a substantial part of the occupational health nurse's role.

Throughout the 1990s there has been a steady growth in the number of community children's nurses. The role of these practitioners has been strengthened by the publications of two reports which support the delivery of integrated care to children across the secondary–primary care interface. The first report, *Flexible Options for Paediatric Care* (British Paediatric Association 1993), sets the scene for the growth in the delivery of secondary care to children, outside of the traditional hospital children's department. There are numerous reasons why this growth has occurred, and these centre around a desire to reduce hospitalization of children, an acceptance by both families and health professionals that home care is preferable, and a blurring of the demarcation between acute and community services. This report was followed in 1996 by the publication of *Child Health in the Community: A Guide to Good Practice* (DoH 1996a). This report was intended to show how the quality and effectiveness of children's services could be improved through the better targeting of resources to families with the greatest need, clearly defining the working relationships between secondary and primary care, and closer collaboration between different organizations responsible for child welfare. While the report did not make specific recommendations, it was designed to raise awareness of good practice amongst commissioners and NHS Trusts. Several organizations worked to make best use of the report to encourage the development of community children's nursing services. The Royal College of Nursing (1996) produced a briefing paper on buying paediatric community nursing for purchasers and commissioners of health care. The paper identified the contribution such practitioners can make to ill children and their families, as well as illustrating how effective, and indeed cost effective, such services could be at reducing in-patient costs and lengths of hospital stay.

Like many other services within the NHS, mental health is undergoing some fundamental changes designed to address some of the problems of the past. In 1998, the government produced proposals to modernize mental health services (Department of Health 1998c). The proposal set out a new vision for the provision of mental health care, which aimed to reduce social exclusion amongst patients with a mental illness, tackle the root causes of mental ill health, and improve services with better assessment, treatment and the support of a modern framework of law. In setting out to reform mental health services the government recognized failures of the past, including inadequate care and services in some areas, underfunding, overburdened carers and an outdated legal framework. Care in the community has failed because, while it improved the treatment of many people who were mentally ill, it left far too many walking the streets, often at risk to themselves and a nuisance to others. A small but significant minority has been a threat to others and themselves (DoH 1998c).

The cornerstones of the new approach are that services will be safe, providing protection for the public and effective care for the patient. Services will be sound, with a full range of easily accessible services being provided. Finally, services will be supportive with more joint working and carer support. Concerns about aspects of the proposals have been voiced, and these centre on the right to detain people, and the nature and scope of compulsion. While the government regard the reforms as promoting social inclusion, these aspects of policy may effectively further socially exclude individuals. The danger is that people, fearing compulsion, will not seek assistance at all when their mental health deteriorates.

The proposals to modernize mental health care are underpinned by new investment to provide extra beds of all kinds, including better outreach services, and 24-hour crisis teams. Service equity will be achieved through the implementation of a new National Service Framework for Mental Health (DoH 1999e). This framework sets the national standards and defines service models for mental health in five key areas. The key areas are mental health promotion, primary care and the access to services, effective services for severe mental illness, caring about carers and preventing suicide. National Service Frameworks will play a major role in shaping the delivery of health care by all health professionals well into the next millennium. Taken together with other government initiatives, such as the National Institute of Clinical Excellence and the Commission for Health Improvement, the future development of clinical practice and services may be clearly mapped out for many practitioners.

At the same time as the modernization of mental health services, the government has set in train a review of the Mental Health Act. The government recognizes that the Mental Health Act has failed to provide an adequate framework for dealing with a quite different group of people: those with severe anti-social personality disorders who present a risk to the public. The main focus of the 1983 Mental Health Act was the compulsory assessment and treatment of patients in hospital. The provision of care has moved on, and it is now widely acknowledged that the legislation is unable to offer sufficient flexibility for the delivery of care outside of hospital. The Department of Health (1999f) produced a consultation document on the reform of the Mental Health Act. Within this document, there are clear proposals for the establishment of compulsion. If approved, the new Act would allow health professionals to apply for a compulsory assessment or treatment order. This would allow for the provision of compulsory care by community based teams without the need for the hospitalization.

The proposed changes within mental health services will result in major change over the next few years. Community psychiatric nurses may find that the teams in which they work will be integrated with secondary care providers. This move is an attempt to ensure that patients, discharged from hospital, are not missed and are provided with the right level of ongoing support. The establishment of 24-hour crisis teams will also result in changes to working patterns, and may offer many opportunities for community staff to be involved in the delivery of acute care. The government has placed responsibility for implementing the new National Service Framework on health authorities and Primary Care Groups, and they also see the need for closer cooperation between specialist mental health services and primary care. This will present many opportunities and challenges from the practitioners involved, as integration of mental health services into primary health care teams has often proved problematic in the past.

◯ Societal changes

A number of changes have taken place within society that have impacted on the day to day working lives of community nurses. Many of these changes, such as the type of employment people undertake, have been discussed earlier in the chapter. Indeed, some of these changes, such as the rising rates of marital breakdown, have led directly to new government initiatives and policy. In just one generation, the rate of first-time marriages has halved, while the divorce rate has trebled. In 1987, there were 260,459 first-time marriages (both partners). This had fallen to 181,135 in the 10 years to 1997 (Office for National Statistics 2000). This, in turn, has directly impacted on the work role of health visitors and school nurses, with more families being headed by single parents, and many children experiencing the breakdown of their parents' marriage. Additionally, the rising rates of teenage pregnancy and efforts to reduce this have impacted on the work of several community practitioners. The proportion of teenagers becoming pregnant fell during the 1970s, but started rising again in the 1980s. Since 1990 the teenage conception rate has fallen to 63 per 1000 in 1996 (Office for National Statistics 1999). Additionally, just under half of all conceptions in under-16s result in maternity, and while teenage birth rates are dropping, the rate of abortion is increasing (Office for National Statistics 1999).

Other changes, such as longer life expectancy, and the growing numbers of elderly people have placed considerable pressure on a whole range of health services. In 1998, there were just over 9 million people aged over 65 in the UK. By 2021, it is estimated that this will have risen to over 12 million (Office for National Statistics 2000). District nurses are often involved in the delivery of continuing nursing care to many of these people who live at home or in residential care, and this is placing services under increasing pressure. The recent Audit Commission report (Audit Commission 1999a) suggests that community trusts should ensure that they have systems in place for monitoring caseload sizes and workloads, as well as specific referral criteria for district nursing interventions.

Since the early 80s there has been an expansion in the range and scope of services available for community care. This has resulted in a change in perception amongst the public about how long term care is provided. The philosophy of care in the community has impacted on all primary care practitioners, resulting in an expansion of nursing support for children, as well as people with mental health problems and learning disabilities. However, several high profile cases, where family carers and members of the public have been attacked or murdered by people with mental health problems (BBC 1998) has resulted in a backlash against care in the community policies. The proposed reform to the Mental Health Act (DoH 1999f), and the modernization of mental health services are part of the government's reaction to this problem.

Finally, changes in the structure of employment have produced profound effects on the health and well-being of employees. The last 30 years have seen the closure of many heavy industries, for example mining and ship building. These industries have been replaced with a growth in manufacturing and service industries. These changes to the nature of employment have resulted in more women entering employment, which can alter family structures, and place increased pressure on family life. All of these changes mean that occupational health nurses see less physical injuries and deaths, but there are now higher levels of stress and mental health problems in the workplace than in previous years.

◯ Conclusion

Understanding how contextual factors can impact on the development of practice is a vitally important part of both deciding what to develop, and how any development might be achieved. Often practitioners have a lack of understanding of how they can use policy to affect local development, and occasionally practitioners can even identify developments that are in conflict with national or local priorities. Such developments are unlikely to succeed because of a lack of commitment and resources. While policy may not be the most important contextual factor, it is probably the most influential. Most national policy initiatives attract resources, either from government or local sources. Policy initiatives are also closely monitored by the Health Departments, and as a result they are very difficult to ignore. By their very nature, policy focused developments are nearly always top-down, and they often involve very prescriptive and directive implementation and operational criteria. Occasionally it is possible for practitioners to initiate a development which fits with the national agenda. Recent examples include the establishment of rapid response teams in mental health, and the running of specialist services providing general health care for people with learning disabilities.

Invariably policy is developed and amended as a result of changes in society. Even the various NHS restructuring exercises have been designed to increase efficiency because of concerns about rising costs associated with demographic change. Furthermore, public pressure as a result of waiting lists has also resulted in a number of changes, including increased rates of day surgery. The structure and the expectations of society can have a profound effect on local service delivery. It is not uncommon for health visitors, working in new towns with high numbers of young children, to have little capacity to do anything other than concentrate on children and families. As society changes, the way in which health care is provided needs to change. The establishment of NHS Direct and walk-in centres are two high profile developments that are designed to meet changes in working patterns and provide health advice and care to individuals who find the traditional general practice with its restrictive appointment times no longer meets their needs for health care.

The final part of this contextual loop relates to how the professions respond to the need for change. It is somewhat inevitable that the professions will be reactive rather than proactive to the need for change. Often it is not until the policy has been developed, that the professions are able to identify the need for change. There are numerous examples of this, including the need for standards related to the educational preparation of nurse practitioners, something which remains to this day several years behind the actual development in practice. As a result there is a wide variation in the skills and knowledge of these practitioners. However, other changes within the nursing profession such as the development of the scope of professional practice guidance, have gone a long way to enabling the development of clinical practice without the constant need for a position statement from the profession. Other changes, such as the implementation of nurse prescribing, were developed by the Health Departments in collaboration with the National Boards for Nursing, Midwifery and Health Visiting. Understanding the factors that drive development is fundamental for any practitioner who wishes to be at the forefront of practice development. Failure to recognize and utilize such drivers will result in problems with both planning and implementation.

② Evidence for development

Charlotte L. Clarke and John Unsworth

◯ Chapter summary

In this chapter we propose to explore the issues around the identification of evidence to support the development of practice. It is not our aim to rehearse the arguments around evidence-based practice, as this has been more than adequately covered in other texts (see for example Muir Gray 1997). Rather, we intend to explore the relationship between sources of knowledge for practitioners and the type of evidence available to the practitioner who intends to develop their practice. Much of the literature exploring evidence-based practice has contrived to make it synonymous with not only 'research-based practice', but research based upon the 'gold standard' randomized controlled trial (RCT). This has resulted in practitioners being bombarded with workshops and courses to equip them with critical appraisal skills and the exhortation from policymakers to enhance research capacity within health organizations. However, it needs to be questioned as to whether all these edicts address the important issues for practitioners wishing to improve patient care. Within this chapter, we will also discuss the sources and types of knowledge practitioners may draw upon to develop their practice.

◯ Introduction

The move towards evidence-based practice is undeniably long overdue. However the issue central to the debate for practitioners is not just how to critique this evidence, but where the evidence comes from, and then how it might be relevant within the context of their own practice.

Despite the move towards evidence-based practice, there has been very little debate about the whole notion of evidence in terms of whether the difference between evidence and research is purely semantic, or whether there is more than one legitimate source of evidence on which to base practice. To open up the discussion about sources of evidence, let us look at Joan's story (Box 2.1). Joan's story does not follow the accepted pathway of evidence-based practice as identified by Sackett *et al.* (1997).

1 formulate an answerable clinical question;
2 locate the best source of evidence to provide an answer to the question;
3 critically appraise the evidence for its validity and usefulness;
4 apply the results of this appraisal to practice;
5 evaluate the outcome.

There are clearly skills required to achieve this pathway to evidence-based practice, such as to find, critically appraise, utilize and evaluate sources of evidence from well-conducted research studies. As can be seen from the example in Box 2.1, Joan drew upon a variety of sources of evidence for this development. The first source of evidence Joan utilized to identify the potential need for development was her own experience of caring for her parents. The use of such forms of evidence is rarely if ever acknowledged, yet it plays a major role in helping us decide what aspects of practice we are interested in developing. It is unlikely that any practitioner will have the same level of interest in every single aspect of their role, and this can often shape the way in which they will introduce or accept changes. While this may not be a significant issue within moderate to large nursing teams such as those often found within district nursing practice, in other areas such as health visiting this reliance on developing those areas of specialist interest could potentially disadvantage certain groups within the community. This suggests that there is a need for groups of practitioners, who have traditionally worked alone, to get together to plan and develop services that go beyond traditional GP practice boundaries, but which provide services to a defined community.

Joan's initial interest in the topic of carers who are children stimulated her to gather evidence of need from within her own practice area. This was achieved through health needs analysis and the identification of those children who were acting as carers within the schools for which Joan was responsible. Once this stage was completed, Joan was able to use published work and her own experience to identify how she was going to develop practice to meet those unmet needs. Finally, evidence of the effectiveness of the package was obtained, using evaluative research and gaining service users' views.

Box 2.1 Joan's story

Joan, 56, has been a school nurse for the last 10 years. In that time, there have been many changes to the nature of her work, all of which have proven to be very challenging. Joan came to nursing late in life after spending many years caring for her parents. When she first qualified, Joan worked on a neurology ward and, after three years, Joan obtained a job in school nursing. Joan recently commenced her Community Health Care studies degree and, as part of her course, she was required to complete a health needs assessment of the area in which she worked. While discussing this project with the headmaster of a large comprehensive school, the problem of children as carers was raised, particularly in relation to attendance and attainment. Joan quickly became engaged with this idea, as it was very dear to her heart. Also it had struck her on a number of occasions, working on the neurology ward, that there were many patients in their 30s and 40s who were dependent upon their children to provide much of their care at home.

As a result of this conversation, Joan set about exploring the scope of the problem. Having completed a needs analysis within the schools she was attached to, it soon became apparent that many children who had identified themselves as carers were missing out, both in their education and social development. Joan was also concerned that what she had uncovered was the tip of the iceberg. Many children did not want to make themselves known to the authorities, as they felt that this would cause trouble for both their parents and themselves. Based upon her academic work, experiential knowledge from her work on neurology, and her own personal experiences, Joan began to develop an assessment package that she and the teachers might be able to use in partnership with the children.

An evaluation of this package after one year demonstrated how important the children found the partnership approach, and also that they and their parents now felt supported. Alongside this evaluation, Joan felt a great deal of satisfaction from her post within the schools, as she now had a role working with the teachers. It had also given her an opportunity to draw upon her past experience and use this within her day to day work.

⊙ Types of evidence for the development of practice

Essentially evidence and its usefulness in developing practice falls into three broad categories. First, evidence may be used to identify the need for development. Typically, most developments have as an antecedent either the awareness of a better way of delivering care or services, or a feeling that the current methods are less than optimal. Evidence of the need for development can come from a number of sources, such as published research, which may highlight deficits in current practice, or from other sources, such as reflection on practice and audit. Some of these sources of evidence will be discussed later in this chapter.

Second, evidence may be used to inform the actual development of practice. In this form, the evidence is used as the basis of change, and it often centres around the development of effective health care. The notion of effectiveness in health care can take many forms, and confusion has often occurred because of a tendency to use terms such as effectiveness, efficiency and efficacy interchangeably. All of these concepts are important in the development of effective practice, and we will discuss each of them in more detail shortly. As an umbrella term, the Department of Health (1996c: 45) defines clinical effectiveness as:

> The extent to which specific clinical interventions, when deployed in the field for a particular patient or population, do what they are intended to do. That is, maintain or improve the health and secure the greatest possible health gain for the resources available.

From this definition it is clear that for any development to be effective, it must not only involve interventions that are based upon evidence indicative of producing the desired outcomes, it must also represent an efficient use of resources. So evidence utilization during the planning and implementation of a development is a vitally important part of the development of practice. Planning a development that has little or no evidence of its effectiveness is likely to lead to failure, principally because of problems accessing resources and gaining approval from managers.

Several areas must be considered when evaluating whether a proposed development is likely to be effective. As highlighted earlier, effectiveness is essentially about whether a particular intervention causes something to happen, which is both observable and measurable. However, clinical effectiveness encompasses much more, including:

- *Efficiency* – Does the output correspond to the level of input? Efficiency in itself does not directly lead to effectiveness; it is, for example, possible to have a very efficient system that is not very effective. A good example would be annual recall for over 75 health checks. The recall system may be very efficient but often the people who come forward for their appointments are those people who are in the least need of intervention. The at-risk elderly people who live alone and are housebound may be completely missed because of the concentration on clinic-based activity.
- *Efficacy* – This term relates to the ability of a specific intervention to produce a desired effect. The term is commonly used in relation to the efficacy of a particular drug.
- *Cost effectiveness* – Cost effectiveness relates to the identification of achieving a unit of effect. For example, if the unit of effect was smoking

cessation, and 20 people embarked upon a six week programme of sessions run by a health visitor, the cost effectiveness of the programme would be judged by calculating the total cost of running the sessions and comparing this with the number of people who stopped smoking. Cost effectiveness of an intervention can be difficult to identify for several reasons. For example, it is often difficult to quantify all of the costs involved, and it may be difficult to identify what costs should be included, for example should travel costs for attendance at the sessions be included? Additionally, when should the outcomes or the effect be measured? In smoking cessation, measuring who had stopped smoking after six weeks is likely to provide a higher rate of stopping than measuring who had stopped one year later.

Third, evidence is generated through the systematic evaluation of developments. This is an important stage in the process of developing practice, as it allows the practitioner to test out both the efficiency and effectiveness of the development, and to identify whether the development is transferable to other areas. Evaluation of practice development is an often neglected stage of the process, and requires considerable skill if it is to be done well. The problematic nature of evaluating developments in practice is discussed later in this chapter.

◯ Identifying areas for development

Fundamental to the effective development of practice is the insight of knowing which areas of practice need to be developed. Research concerns the development of knowledge. However the relationship between the development of practice and undertaking research is not always clear. Research and development are often said in one breath, but to what extent can they be undertaken simultaneously? It is, perhaps, easy to think of developments that have gone ahead without either being based on research evidence or that have not been evaluated to demonstrate their effectiveness. Similarly, it is easy to think of research that has not affected practice. In the health service, we have often divorced research and development, and are now committing a great deal of time and energy in bringing the two together.

Most practitioners, however, even with the most limited skills of critiquing, are able to think of practices that they would wish to see change. This can be thought of as 'grumble power'! Clarke *et al.* (1998) surveyed 219 practitioners who were active in developing practice in one NHS region of England. They found that the main factor that triggered a change in practice was an awareness in the practitioner that the needs of patients were not being met.

Every grumble is a critique of practice, so these should be nurtured rather than contained. Grumbles can arise from:

- a theoretical knowledge that is at odds with practice (this frequently happens when someone studying a course is required to look critically at the literature base of a specific topic);
- a frustration with either practice or their own lack of knowledge and understanding of a clinical issue;
- being asked questions by different people, which suddenly sheds a different light on a situation;
- becoming aware of areas of practice that could be improved, perhaps following an audit, the complaints of patients and relatives, a visit to another clinical area, or participation in a conference or study day.

It is a substantial step, though, to translate a grumble into a practice development or a research project. Not all questions and problems need to be answered by doing research yourself. It may be possible to conduct a literature search, read all the material that is available, and make a decision based on this knowledge, together with your own knowledge of your practice environment. For example, there is perhaps no need to undertake research into the provision of aids to help people take their medication after discharge – it is obvious that such a step should be taken to enable people to take medication successfully and safely.

If, however, you find little to help you decide how to develop practice, then undertaking research may be the way forward, either before implementing any change (to find out more about the nature of the problem for example) or as a built-in part of developing practice, so that you know whether the change is making any difference. Some of the key areas of practice development work that need to involve research activity are in evaluating changes, identifying the perspectives of the users of the service, challenging the professional assumptions of practice, surveying and predicting the outcome of particular forms of intervention. The development of practice is often very fluid and responsive to the developing awareness of the needs of that practice environment. As such, some of the traditional research models may be of limited use, since they emphasize a static, 'outsider' view of services. Some of the action research and participatory action research frameworks may be useful to consider because they allow the simultaneous gathering of data, changing of practice, and questioning of professional roles (for example, Hart and Bond 1995; Meyer and Batehup 1997).

Most often you will be able to use existing evidence or knowledge from the literature to inform your development. The process of applying evidence that has been published in the public domain to a single clinical environment with its own distinct patient and staff population is complex. The merits of the evidence must itself be established, and the implications of 'known evidence' are that it also indicates what it is that we do not know. There seems to be so little research-based evidence that we may conclude, at times, that most of professional practice is beyond the limits of our knowledge. Indeed this is sometimes clearly apparent when evidence becomes a political tool. You may recall the bovine spongiform encephalopathy (BSE) crisis of 1996, when the UK government repeatedly claimed 'there is no evidence to show that the infection can be transmitted to humans'. Indeed there wasn't, but only because this was beyond the limits of our knowledge, which is quite different from having the evidence to show that it *cannot* be transmitted. In a similar way, evidence cannot be separated from beliefs about that which is valued and correct in any society, and it therefore becomes a 'political' tool. Evidence that is inconsistent with society's beliefs will probably never be sought, funded, articulated or disseminated, because it is not near the top of the agenda of research or practice development activity.

In utilizing evidence, there is a growing awareness, then, of this being the edge of not knowing and having no evidence. If everything becomes less certain, how do we develop our practice? Not only is uncertainty uncomfortable, because we do not know whether or not we are doing the correct thing, but we have few indicators of how to develop or even continue our practice. Indeed, if we were to cease all the health and social care practices for which there is no evidence of benefit, what would we have left? Fortunately, this does not mean that these un-proven practices are necessarily wrong, but simply that the evidence for their effectiveness is beyond current knowledge. These are the areas then, where we need to develop the evidence. Until then, practice must continue, based as far as is possible on the principles of care which we may, or may not, all hold to be correct. For example, anything that sup-ports patient autonomy and independence must be good – or must it? Perhaps it is not for those patients intent on self-harm.

One difficult question, when seeking to develop practice, is 'how much evidence is enough?' The answer must vary from one clinical area to another, and from one topic to another. There is, for example, sufficient evidence to advocate the introduction of assessment tools for pressure area care, so long as it is acknowledged that such tools must only sup-plement, and not replace clinical observation and decision making. There is perhaps sufficient evidence to demonstrate the effectiveness of educat-ing patients, pre-discharge, about their post-discharge medication use. However, just what is the purpose of such an intervention? This may be compliance with prescriptions ('follow the instructions' type of educa-tion) or it may be knowledgeable use of medication (when, can and should medications be used or not used, and what are the side-effects?). The evidence needed to demonstrate effectiveness differs in each case.

The context in which the evidence is being applied is also vital. To take the previous example, can you act on the evidence that supports education about medication if your patients all have limited vision or dementia? What else must you do to ensure the safe implementation of the evidence in these situations? Do you have a skill mix that enables this step to be undertaken? Service delivery is dependent on the context and process of change. As Ross and Meerabeau (1997: 5) argue,

> robust evidence on current management of leg ulcer treatment will not produce real health gains, if the factors associated with patient compliance and the organisational issues implicit in the process of care, are not understood.

In these ways, any evidence has to be acknowledged for what it does not tell us, just as much as for what it does tell us. There then needs to be a vital step of applying the evidence to a single clinical environment and the context in which that care is to be delivered.

⬤ The impact of differential knowledge on practice

Just to complicate the picture of evidence further, we need to recognize that there is no single version of understanding an issue. This plurality of knowledge results in several different ways of seeing an issue. We can use the example given in Table 2.1, drawn from dementia care, to illustrate this.

If you wanted to develop services for people with dementia, and you were working within the patho-physiological domain, then you might start a clinic, offering diagnostic screening; you might start a carer education group, and you would be unlikely to offer any health promotion activities to the person with dementia. However, if you wanted to develop services and care, and you were working within the psycho-social domain, you might start a day centre, and offer interventions such as reality orientation and encourage group activities, to help people with dementia stay connected to our 'real world'.

If you wanted to develop care and services and were working within the interactional domain, then you would try to keep the family together, and would want to work with the individual's past life. So you might use life history work or family nursing. You would be less likely to offer day unit care or respite care, but would favour domiciliary support systems. Working within a sociocritical domain, you would be developing care and services that are very rare at present. You would be encouraging the independent living of people with dementia, for example, in supported living environments. You would feel that the opportunity

Table 2.1 Differential knowledge in dementia care (from Clarke 1999a)

Domain	Causality and diagnosis of dementia	Role of health and social care professional
Patho-physiology	Physical cause. Early identification sought as an essential precursor to treatment.	Care focus on needs of family carer. Interventions emphasize 'geriatric routine', containment, pharmaceutical management, carer education and search for a cure.
Psycho-sociological	Physical cause with social and psychological influences. Socially 'different' and cognitively incompetent.	Aim to 'bring back' person with dementia. Interventions emphasize the 'real' world e.g. Reality Orientation.
Interactional	Emphasis on the social creation of dementia. Diagnosis may undermine self and relationships.	Individualized care sought within family context. Interventions emphasize self-validation and life history work.
Social critical	Dementia socially and culturally constructed. Diagnosis may be empowering.	Able to appreciate and work with 'other' realities. Interventions may seek to work with the individuals as active members of social framework e.g. family therapy.

to participate in the local community is important for basic health and well-being. You would also recognize that the needs of people are determined in part by the ability of services and practitioners to deliver care. For example, nobody 'needs' day care, but day care is one of the ways of meeting their need for, say social interaction. Similarly, nobody 'needs' residential or nursing home care, but this is the form of non-domiciliary care that is most prevalent in the UK for those who are not able to sustain living in their own home (although this point of unsustainability is itself determined by the availability and flexibility of services).

Thus we can understand that the way in which we 'see' an issue has a major influence on the way in which we seek to care for people. Furthermore, there are several different views to be understood, and although dementia care has been used as an example here, similar issues apply to most areas of health care.

◯ Sources of knowledge

Having been exhorted to implement research-based practice, there is now a strong national drive to implement evidence-based practice. While this shift in terminology may appear to be one of semantics only, there are some important issues to consider. First, what is the difference between 'research' and 'evidence'? Second, how can we identify 'good' research and 'good' evidence? Third, does evidence always arise from research, or can there be other sources of evidence?

Increasingly, evidence is collated through systematic reviews. A systematic review uses a research strategy to evaluate all research on a specified topic area, and produces recommendations based on the collective message of all this research. Kendall (1997) argues that evidence-based practice implies this thorough evaluation of the evidence, and is therefore more than research-based practice. The recommendations from a systematic review are then disseminated. For example, they are published as clinical guidelines, and in journals such as *Evidence-Based Nursing* or *Evidence-Based Medicine*. Guidelines are produced at both national and local levels and so you may find more than one for a specific clinical topic. For example, guidelines are available for continence care from the US Department of Health and Human Services (1992), the Association for Continence Advice (1993) and the Royal College of Physicians (1995).

Systematic reviews provide a very good way of finding out what the research evidence is for a specific procedure or client group. However, they produce global recommendations, and the synthesis of research findings from a range of studies may lead to unequivocal recommendations that are difficult to relate to your own client group. Reviews also synthesize research results from tightly defined methodologies and rarely combine different types of methodology in one report (such as RCTs and case control studies). Robust methods have been developed for combining findings from randomized controlled trials and these have a greater weighting than other research methodologies. Methods for combining findings from other types of methodologies are still in their infancy. Further, you will need to consider how useful the information is for you, in your own work environment and for your client/patient group. This is what Kendall (1997: 23) calls for when she writes that: 'in order to give the highest quality of care, nurses working in primary care need to consider the meaning of evidence and to draw on evidence arising from different philosophical research positions'.

It may be that it is at this stage you need to draw upon other forms of knowledge. This may be the knowledge that you have gained by working as a practitioner: experiential knowledge. This form of knowledge allows you to know of another form of evidence that is specific to your own context of care delivery. This is exactly the situation in which Joan, in the earlier case study, found herself.

A third form of evidence arises from a knowledge of theoretical issues, for example in understanding the potential stigma associated with drug abuse, mastectomy or stoma care. In addition, your knowledge may be informed by certain beliefs and values. For example, fundamental issues about practice are governed by a strong belief that life is valuable and people are individuals.

There are, therefore, at least four sources of evidence that can be drawn on in practice: research, experiential, theoretical, beliefs and values. There is a need to juggle these different forms of evidence in deciding how and when to develop practice.

At times, it is important to exclude some evidence as inappropriate. Most often, this happens when a piece of evidence becomes out of date. It may also happen when one form of evidence is in conflict with another form of evidence. For example, the research and experiential evidence may indicate the benefits of a blood transfusion, but your beliefs and values may allow you to respect someone's wish to decline a transfusion. In this case, some evidence becomes inappropriate for the context of that patient's care.

There is a need to think about the extent to which evidence is political, or is used politically. A quick scan through a selection of daily newspapers, produces some interesting items. For example, in 1996 publicity to promote the work of the Nutrition Task Force was reported to have been blocked following protests from the food industry, and the *Daily Mail* of 25 November 1997 reported a watering-down of the powers of the Food Standards Agency, to oversee the nutritional content of food.

Many developments in practice have arisen from policy directives, for example the care of older people, and those with mental health needs, has been dramatically altered following the Community Care Act (DoH 1990). It is not always clear what evidence there is for such policies, and yet their impact on practice is widespread and sometimes irreversible. Similarly, at times, the policies available do not reflect the dynamic nature of knowledge development. For example, Mulhall (1995: 580) writes that: 'Health policy does not automatically adjust to the changing knowledge base of nursing'.

None the less, evidence-based practice has assumed a great deal of importance in developing practice. It is not sufficient to base practice on the obvious or the tried and tested. Although these may well be appropriate actions, they must have a robust body of knowledge that supports their effectiveness. Then not only can effective care be demonstrable, but also it can continue to be developed as an understanding of how and why a particular intervention works and evolves.

There is a need to differentiate between evidence that can be applied to anyone in any context (in other words it is generalizable from the study sample to a larger population), and which is usually developed by carefully controlled clinical trials, and evidence that is derived from a local knowledge of the patient group and health care delivery services. Both are important but for different reasons. Just as it is wrong to graft evidence onto an inappropriate clinical environment, it is wrong to ignore either type of evidence altogether.

There are a variety of criteria by which a piece of evidence may be judged. Some which you may like to consider are whether the evidence:

- is research-based (rather than an anecdotal account);
- is defined for a specific context (where, and for which patients etc., is the evidence appropriate);
- has had a clear and demonstrable impact on patient outcomes (bearing in mind whether the criteria for such outcomes are appropriate and for whom);
- is valid (was the way in which the evidence was established based on appropriate criteria that can be applied elsewhere);
- is generalizable (can you use the evidence directly, or does it make you think about your own practice – the latter is sometimes known as catalytic validity);
- is practice or theoretical knowledge (what is the source of knowledge which informs the evidence, or ideally, does it draw on both practice and theory);
- has a breadth of relevance (what are the limits of the relevance of the knowledge for patient groups, staff groups, clinical areas etc. as well as over time).

When collecting information and putting together a case for a development, it is important to use knowledge in a balanced way – both in terms of the source of that knowledge and the selectivity of it. For example, a good proposal will have a balance of research-based evidence, together with a statement about why it is important for your organization and your client group, which draws more heavily on an experiential knowledge base. In addition, the research-based evidence presented should be a summary of all that is known about a topic, not a one-sided story. So avoid pulling out selected publications that support your point of view, whilst ignoring all the other publications that agree less strongly with your plans.

One of the major disadvantages of using evidence derived from a literature or research base is that it may squeeze out the voice of the service user themselves. Part of the reason for this is the emphasis that society places on technical knowledge, so that lay versions of health and illness are valued less than medical knowledge. A second reason is that we have poorly developed mechanisms for accessing service users' views (unlike research evidence with its network of publications, libraries and clinical guidelines). Service users rarely have a single voice that is heard loudly. Following on from this is a third reason for service users to be disadvantaged – the voice that professional staff are most likely to hear is that of the white middle classes and middle aged. Consequently we need to be cautious about accepting their views as representative of all service users; indeed, it is more likely that social inequalities will be perpetuated.

However there are a number of ways in which you can and should use service user perspectives. If you feel through your experiential knowledge that the needs of service users are not being fully met, you may do some research to find out the scale and nature of the problem. This could range from a simple survey to a major piece of qualitative research to help you conceptualize the needs of service users. You may have implemented a change in practice (possibly based on research evidence) and need to evaluate whether service users feel it meets their desired outcomes. You may be part of a developing service that is offering a different type of care to people, and need to understand what impact the new service has on their quality of life, and whether the new service is really helping or simply pushing the problem on to another agency or the family.

User perspectives research can be used to inform the development of practice through the identification of need. This type of evidence can prove very powerful in convincing colleagues and managers of the need for change. Additionally, it can assist with the planning of service provision, allowing for the development of efficient services, which users desire. This is illustrated in Hazel's story (Box 2.2).

Hazel's story clearly shows the importance of user involvement in both identifying the need for development, and planning the nature of future service provision. Hazel experienced uncomfortable feelings about the way in which adolescents were receiving out-patient care alongside other younger children, and this provided the initial trigger for considering developing practice. While the paediatrician did not see this as a problem, he was keen to be involved in the care of older patients with cystic fibrosis. This demonstrates that different professionals may have different driving forces underpinning their desire to develop practice. Identifying these driving forces is an important role for the change facilitator, because without an understanding of these, the implementation of a development may be fraught with difficulty, and resistance from staff is likely to be high. The selling of an idea is an important aspect of developing practice; this is discussed in more depth in Chapter 3.

It is always valuable to remember that any knowledge base is incomplete. Indeed, a knowledge base tells us as much about what we don't

---

Box 2.2   Hazel's story

Since I came into post as a community children's nurse, I was involved in Professor Thompson's cystic fibrosis (CF) clinic. The clinic runs each week, on a Thursday morning and has a wide age range of attenders. One thing which has always struck me is that you can have people in their late teens and babies attending the same clinic. I had voiced my concerns on several occasions, about whether this was indeed the best environment for adolescents to voice their concerns or raise issues about their illness. Indeed, I had discussed my concerns with Professor Thompson on several occasions, but he had stated that he didn't think it was too much of a problem because people were seen individually within a clinic room.

One day, while walking between ward blocks I met Colin, a former patient of Professor Thompson's, who was now in his early 20s. He was now under the care of Dr Saunders, the respiratory physician, and had just attended the main out-patient department. Colin told me that he missed the highly specialized attention of Professor Thompson, as he now attended a general chest clinic. During our next clinic, I told Professor Thompson about my encounter with Colin, and he told me that he had always felt that there was a need for a specialist CF clinic for adults. I asked him if he had ever shared his view with the Trust, but he said that, without evidence, this would simply fall upon deaf ears. I asked if we could not do some work to gather the evidence to support this idea. To my surprise, Professor Thompson agreed.

Over the next three months we set about running focus groups and collecting data on the number of adolescents and adults with CF. The focus groups in particular provided powerful evidence of the need to develop a new way of delivering the services currently provided. Professor Thompson and I were both surprised by the responses we received from patients.

Once we had all of the data together, we went to the Trust board to present our findings, together with an option appraisal of possible ways forward. The Trust board agreed with our plan to re-engineer the existing services so that an adolescent and adult CF service could be provided.

---

know, as what we do know. This is essential, since it helps us to determine priorities for future research. However, 'not knowing' is obviously problematic in practice, and results in a patchwork of knowledge about care that has holes in it. The fragmentation of knowledge perpetuates a task orientated interpretation of health and social care practice (Kendall 1997). For example, interpersonal communication models have been promoted through pre-qualifying education programmes and others, yet this reductionalist approach (such as maintain eye contact, sit at the same level) obscures the context of that communication as being within a practitioner–client relationship, to the detriment of its therapeutic potential.

There is a lack of knowledge about some quite fundamental issues concerning dementia care, for example. One issue is that of the relationship between practitioners and family carers and the person with dementia (Clarke 1999b; Lyons and Zarit 1999), and this lack of knowledge has resulted in care interventions that have been unknowingly abusive of the relationship between the person with dementia and their carer (Carter 1999). Most often, this abuse has resulted from assumptions of involvement, based on gender and kin relationships (e.g. Ungerson 1987). Carers who are spouses have been exploited by policies and practices that have failed to recognize the tensions in a relationship that is both caregiving and marital (Carter 1999).

In summary, there are a number of different ways of securing the knowledge to support the development of practice – none of which are entirely straightforward, of course. There is a large body of existing knowledge available in books and papers and based on theoretical frameworks or empirical research. This must be used appropriately, and the process of applying such knowledge to your own clinical context is complex. There is also a need to recognize that service users do not have an equal voice with practitioners or a written knowledge base, and we do need to find mechanisms to protect and amplify their messages.

◯ Mechanisms to support the development of practice

Integral to the development and advancement of clinical practice is the need to articulate the impact that any development has had, and the need to collect information to support a development in the first place. Some of the main ways in which this is achieved include evaluation, research, audit and structured reflection.

Evaluation

Evaluation can be an important source of evidence where a new way of working has been tried as part of a pilot, or where the practitioner is planning to introduce a development that was initiated within a different practice setting. Evaluative research is a very large subarea of research designs, and is quite complicated when trying to evaluate something as evolving and organic as practice development. Phillips *et al.* (1994: 1) describe evaluation as: 'usually attempt[ing] to measure the extent to which certain *outcomes* can be validly correlated with *inputs* and/or *outputs*. The aim is to establish whether there is a cause–effect relationship'. Evaluations may be traditionally undertaken by an external researcher who has not been involved in (and therefore been 'contaminated' by) any of the development work. One example of a standard evaluation design, compares post-intervention measures with pre-intervention measures using pre-identified criteria. Phillips *et al.* (1994) provide a very readable overview of evaluation methods. Conventional evaluation models may work and be appropriate for practice developments, but may well be problematic.

First, who is best suited to undertake the evaluation? Perhaps obviously, it needs to be someone with a knowledge of research strategies, who is therefore able to design an evaluation study, collect and understand research data. But do they also need to have a knowledge of the practice environment? This 'insider' knowledge which a practitioner knows may be of vital importance in making decisions about what data is important to collect, why and how. Practitioners who have been involved with the development may be seen to be too subjective however, and lack the presumed quality of objectivity in evaluating the development. This is a large debate that is important to consider without any assumptions about which is 'better' (Clarke and Procter 1999). Practitioners who have been involved in a development may also have a strong sense of ownership of the development, and be wary of an 'outsider' coming to examine their work.

Second, a decision needs to be made about what it is that is being evaluated. This may either focus on the outcomes of the development, and ideally the patient outcomes, or the processes of having undertaken the development, for example shifts of power and negotiation. The evaluation may consider both of these. It is important to think about who is setting the criteria for evaluation, as every party may want something slightly different out of it: cost effectiveness vs cost reduction vs professional role development vs patient independence vs family involvement in care and so on. It is surprisingly easy to mix up outcomes for ourselves as professionals and our service, with outcomes for the client. One way of demonstrating this is to ask yourself and your colleagues what is a 'good day'. Now ask what is a 'good day' for your service users, but double check – is this what they really think is a good day, or what you think should be a good day for them? For example, when these questions were asked of a group of social workers and community psychiatric nurses caring for people with enduring mental health needs, the practitioners felt a good day for them was one that ran smoothly. They felt a good day for their service users was to be alive at the end of the day – but arguably, this is an imposition of a professionally defined outcome; the service users themselves unfortunately may consider being alive at the end of the day a less than desirable option.

Further, the timing of establishing evaluation criteria and their flexibility is crucial. Because a development of practice is quite fluid, it would not be surprising if the aims of the development evolved such that criteria established predevelopment would become inappropriate later on. If used, the original criteria would fail to capture the effectiveness of the development, but if criteria are changed, the opportunity for demonstrating an improvement in outcomes would be lost.

Some evaluation designs require you to be able to attribute changes to the new intervention, so that you can say with confidence that the new intervention brought about changes in specified outcomes. However in health care, this amount of control over cause and effect can be very difficult to achieve and there are probably many other factors that have influenced the outcomes. For example, changes in the level of incontinence in a nursing home may be improving because of your education of the nursing home staff. However, they may be also improving because the home has started to take less dependent residents, who are less likely to be incontinent.

Another example, the introduction of clinical supervision in community nursing to improve patient care, may appear to be straightforward. It is fairly easy to measure whether staff are actually receiving supervision, and indeed, it may also be possible to identify the quality of that supervision (for example, through direct observation or secondary data, such as supervision records). However, if we recall that the purpose of the supervision was to improve the quality of patient care, the nature of the evaluation becomes much more problematic. Even if we measure quality using an assessment tool before and after establishing clinical supervision, it would be almost impossible to attribute any change in quality directly to supervision.

Third, the need to evaluate any development needs to be anticipated. All too often a change is implemented, seems to work and then more systematic information is sought to prove its effectiveness. This approach to evaluation fails to capture the vital pre-change data, which is needed to demonstrate any improvement as a result of the development. However, can the pre-change state be anticipated, as even to plan a change will have resulted in an increased awareness of the issue and changes in the practitioners involved? Furthermore, there is a need to develop evaluation strategies that will not delay the implementation of a change, if that change is well supported by an evidence base. There is a limit to how many times something needs to be 'proved' to work, but there is also a need to consider its effectiveness in a specific patient care area.

In Chapter 3, the desire within the NHS for rapid results, often as a consequence of management restructuring and instability, is identified as a factor that may influence the development of practice. This often has a negative influence, not least because it can force a change without thorough planning, which may increase resistance from practitioners. In addition, the desire for rapid results may also have a negative impact on evaluation, because the same forces that drove the development require that any evaluation also be conducted rapidly. Evaluating a new post or service, say within six months of inception, may fail to recognize the lead-in time for development. Take for example, the establishment of a new clinic or group session – it will take several months before the number of referrals reaches the level of subsequent functioning of the service. Most often, an evaluation looks at the phase of development rather than the subsequent phase of maintenance or sustained functioning, and these are two very different phases in the life of a development.

Fourth, the methods of evaluation will need to be chosen, either by an external evaluator or by the practitioners themselves. Key questions are about collecting the right data, which will enable potential effectiveness to be demonstrated and which will acknowledge how diverse and fluid the impact of change may be. For example, early discharge may reduce waiting lists, but also affect the quality of that experience for patients. Evaluation using the former criteria will miss half the impact of the development. Alternatively, it may be quite some time before the full impact of an intervention is realized. Health promotion activity is a classic area that has problems here, with outcome evaluations undertaken after a short period of time, revealing little more than uncertain or incomplete outcomes.

Often audit departments are approached to help with evaluations of developments, but there is a need to consider how appropriate the audit process is for demonstrating some forms of change, since they often emphasize the quantitative, measurable aspects of practice. Methods that involve integrating evaluation and development, such as action research (for example Birkett 1995; Meyer and Batehup 1997), and those undertaken by the people involved in the development, such as participatory research (Cornwall and Jewkes 1995), are gaining greater acceptance in the research world.

A crucial part of selecting evaluation methods is consideration of a range of ethical issues. Several ethical principles are important in any practice development, including non-maleficence (the duty to do no harm) and beneficence (the duty to do good). These ethical principles have a major impact on how you might decide to do an evaluation. For example, you may be introducing better systems of bereavement care, but follow-up interviews after someone has died may be inappropriate. Or you may feel that patients are agreeing too readily to participate in the evaluation because their consent is not fully informed, or because they see you as a helpful nurse, rather than an evaluator. You will certainly need to think through how to manage patient confidentiality, anticipating dilemma situations that demand that, as a practitioner, you act on information (for example, an interview may lead you to think that someone is being abused) although you have given assurances of confidentiality as a researcher.

Research

Numerous authors have described the importance of research in the identification of the need to develop practice. While this may be one of the most widely referred to forms of evidence in practice, it is often underutilized. Greenwood (1984) and Rolfe (1996) suggest that scientific knowledge has had very little influence upon nursing practice. There are several reasons why this might occur.

1 *Dissemination* – Obviously the way in which research findings are disseminated to practitioners will have an impact upon their subsequent use in practice. Current methods of dissemination often cause problems with awareness, access and interpretation, and all of this contributes to the theory–practice gap in nursing (Dickson 1996a). One of the principal problems with dissemination of research is that it is often diffused rather than disseminated. While dissemination is meant to be active and very targeted, diffusion implies a more general passage of information, which may be untargeted and haphazard. As a result, the research findings may not reach their intended target audience. This problem is further compounded by the fact that research is often published in academic journals. Publication in this type of journal brings academic kudos and assists academic institutions to meet the demands of the research assessment exercise, but this results in it being less accessible to the practitioner.

2 *Problems with access* – Droogan and Song (1996: 15) suggest that 'practitioners involved in patient care rarely have the time, resources and skills to gather together and critically appraise relevant research in an effort to inform their practice'. Clearly the problems of access to research findings and published literature are ever present for most nurses. However, the geographical isolation of many areas of community practice means that these problems are further compounded. The move of nurse education into higher education has resulted in the relocation of many nursing libraries away from the workplace, onto an often distant campus. In some cases, access has been further restricted by the withdrawal of borrowing rights from NHS staff who are not studying with the higher education provider. The NHS has struggled to provide resources of a similar calibre, although a great deal of work has taken place developing electronic resources. Such resources are particularly welcome for staff working in primary care, who may practice many miles from a hospital or higher education library.

3 *Lack of understanding or fear* – Despite the fact that research methods are an integral part of many nurse education programmes, many practitioners experience problems in understanding the methodology and results of studies (Hunt 1984). Wallis (1998: 6) describes how 'it appears that generating research data is not enough to influence practice.

Practitioners lack the knowledge, skills and attitudes to integrate research into their care'. Problems in understanding research studies mean that many nurses are fearful of using original studies as the basis for developing practice. Mulhall (1995) describes how 'contradictory results and explanations, which evolve from different studies, present a problem for the practising nurse who needs unambiguous solutions to practical problems'. There are several ways in which research can be translated into usable forms, including the development of clinical practice guidelines, the use of which will be described shortly. Firstly, let us look at another issue related to the use of research in practice, that of translation.

4 *Translation problems* – Some of the evidence produced through traditional forms of research will not be presented in a clinically useful form. Brett (1987) describes this as not being 'practice ready'. The lack of clinical application in some studies results in problems for the practitioner, in trying to decide what it is that needs to change. A great deal of the evidence produced by researchers may need considerable analysis before its significance to practice can be determined (Bircumshaw 1990).

The distance between evidence in the form of research and how practitioners practice can be minimized by using approaches such as practitioner and action research. Such approaches can have a significant impact on practice because they allow for the study of issues that are unique to the local practice area. Action research consists of a cyclical series of activities, which include the examination of a local issue or problem, gathering data to solve that problem, implementing change and gathering further data to monitor and evaluate the impact of the change. Hart and Bond (1995) describe how action research should be context related and collaborative, involving both change and theory generation. The use of such approaches to research are not without their problems. Such problems include the conflict between being a practitioner and being a researcher. For example, one consequence is the difficulty of analysing data without applying the pre-existing lens of a professional background (Reed and Procter 1995).

However research evidence can be presented in different forms that are much more user friendly. Systematic reviews, for example, provide a comprehensive overview of the research produced on a particular topic. A good systematic review should provide the practitioner with an indication of the best intervention, or enough evidence for the practitioner to combine the evidence that is available, with clinical judgement so that practice can be developed. Dickson (1996a: 8) states 'the availability of a good systematic review should increase the nurses' confidence in the research findings, as well as guiding their implementation'. The availability of systematic reviews has increased in recent years, thanks in part to the development of specialist centres such as the Cochrane Collaboration and the NHS Centre for Reviews and Dissemination (NHS CRD). While the more widespread availability of such evidence is welcomed, practitioners may still experience problems in translating the findings of a review into evidence for the development of practice. A clear example is the review published on the treatment of head lice and scabies (NHS CRD 1999). This review suggested that there was little or no evidence that the 'wet combing' method was effective. Some practitioners misinterpreted this to mean that this method was ineffective, whereas in fact the method had not at the time been subjected to a controlled trial to measure its effectiveness.

Guidelines are a useful method of overcoming some of the problems associated with the translation of evidence into a practice-ready format. The need to provide evidence in a form useful to practitioners, together with the reduction in variations in practice, has provided the impetus for the development of such guidelines. Additional driving forces have included rising health costs and the potential for increased litigation (Dickson 1996b).

Woolf (1990: 1811) defines clinical practice guidelines as 'official statements of policies from major organisations and agencies on the proper indications for performing a procedure or treatment or the proper management of a specific clinical problem'. Essentially, there are four methods of developing clinical practice guidelines:

- *Informal consensus* is based upon the opinion of experts. While this approach often involves the use of evidence in the form of published literature and expert opinion, there is little guarantee that the evidence sources will be comprehensive and unbiased.
- *Formal consensus* is based upon the opinion of an expert panel who meet to discuss a particular issue. This approach is often used where the research evidence is inconclusive, but there is a need to produce some guidelines for continued practice.
- *Evidence-based guideline development* is based upon an unbiased systematic review of the evidence. The review is usually conducted to a clear protocol and will include published and unpublished (grey) literature.
- *Explicit guideline development* goes beyond the use of evidence, as it usually specifies the benefits, harms and costs of interventions, as well as establishing the probability of achieving the desired outcomes.

Guidelines can provide the trigger to develop practice by presenting the evidence for development in an easily accessible form. Despite the benefits of guidelines, it is important to remember that the process of actually developing practice remains the responsibility of the practitioner. In some cases, the required developments are easy to achieve,

Box 2.3   Elaine's story

After three years as a relief district nursing sister, I was really looking forward to my new job, attached to Dr McCullach and partners. I was replacing Margo Bavostock, who had just retired. Margo and her staff nurse had worked in the practice for 12 years, following the amalgamation of two smaller practices. My appointment corresponded with the publication of the SIGN (Scottish Inter-collegiate Network) guidelines on the treatment and management of leg ulceration. This is an area I was particularly interested in, and I had already completed a short course in leg ulcer management.

I set about reviewing the documentation and reassessing the patients on the caseload as necessary. I was struck by the fact that none of the patients with leg ulcers had ever had their ankle brachial pressure index (ABPI) measured. Some of the patients were even having compression bandages applied, even though we did not know for definite that their ulcers were indeed venous. Over the next four days, I visited all of the patients and reassessed them. Luckily, the patients receiving compression did indeed have venous ulcers, although I remained concerned about whether the bandages were being applied correctly. Wilma, the staff nurse, did not know how to measure a patient's ABPI. So I provided her with instruction and let her measure a new patient's ABPI over the next few weeks. Additionally, we undertook joint visits, so I could instruct her about bandaging and assess her competence.

Working together, Wilma and I were able to adapt our practice so that we were following the SIGN guidelines, and this in turn led to improvements in the care we were able to provide to patients. This was demonstrated by the fact that, over a two month period, four patients had their ulcers completely healed.

as illustrated in Elaine's story (Box 2.3), but other aspects of practice may prove more problematic because they involve the introduction of change across several disciplines.

Elaine's story illustrates the use of evidence-based guidelines to develop practice. There were several triggers for this development. First, Elaine was interested in the area of practice to be developed. As highlighted earlier, initial interest in an aspect of practice is an important driving force behind most developments. Unless a practitioner is interested in a particular topic, they are unlikely to spend time examining the evidence about a particular intervention.

The second trigger behind the development was the review of the documentation that took place after Elaine came into post. This review identified deficits in the care delivered to patients and highlighted potential risks associated with current practice, for example, the application of compression without a vascular assessment.

Finally, the publication of the SIGN guidelines was another major trigger. These guidelines supplied Elaine with a succinct and usable review of the evidence related to the care of patients with leg ulceration. Using the guidelines, Elaine was able to identify which aspects of practice needed to be improved, and she set about improving these through better documentation and clinical teaching for her colleague.

The development of practice using the guidelines was fairly simple in this case because it only involved a small and motivated team of practitioners. In areas where other nurses were involved, this could have proven problematic. Take, for example, a situation where leg ulcers are cared for by both the district nursing team and the practice nurses. Improving care in this scenario becomes much more complicated, because it involves different groups of staff. The practice nurses are unlikely to be employed by the same people as the district nurses, and this can create problems in trying to introduce change. Clearly, strategies involving power will be of little use in this situation and change can only be effectively brought about through negotiation and re-education.

Audit

Clinical audit can be a major source of evidence for the development of practice. Audit can be used either to identify areas where practice needs to develop, or to evaluate small scale developments before their wider roll-out within an organization. Garland and Corefield (1999: 130) state that 'audit provides confirmation of the consistent application of best practice, or reveals practice that is not consistent and ineffective'. While audit had existed within the NHS for a number of years, its use became more widespread following the publication of *Working for Patients* (DoH 1989). Initially audit was concerned about the measurement of standards of care, but more recently it has moved on to include notions of effective practice. Clinical audit is described as:

> a clinically led initiative, which seeks to improve the quality and outcome of patient care through structured peer review, whereby clinicians examine their practices and results against agreed explicit standards, and modify their practice, where indicated.
>
> (NHS Executive 1996b: 3)

Many writers have compared clinical audit and research (Balogh 1996). While there are a number of similarities, especially related to the methods of data collection used, audit differs from research in a number of ways. The most important of these is, that while research is concerned with identifying the 'right thing to do', audit is about ensuring 'the right things are, in fact, done' (Balogh 1996).

Box 2.4   Marion's story

Both my colleagues and I had operated an internal rotation system, providing 24-hour cover within a large car assembly plant. While night duty provided less opportunity for health promotion activity, it was no less busy, with a number of employees needing attention for accidental injuries. The shift system operated by the occupational health nursing team meant that it was more difficult to identify a pattern of injury rates between the different shifts. However, during a conversation over coffee one day, my colleague Claire remarked that we were substantially busier on the fifth night before the shift changed over.

Claire and I decided to instigate an audit of injuries over the last year, to identify if there was a pattern associated with the duration of night shifts. The audit revealed that accidental injury was more common during nights four and five, and the incident reports appeared to suggest that employee error was a significant contributing factor to many of these injuries.

Claire and I presented our audit findings to the operational management board of the plant, and they agreed to consider possible solutions to reduce the duration of night shifts. After several months of negotiations with the workforce and unions, the plant eventually adopted a new four-shift system, making the night shift significantly shorter. This will, hopefully, have the effect of making employees less tired and thereby reducing accidental injury.

Audit can be a powerful trigger in the development of practice. Often, the trigger is the provision of feedback to individual practitioners and others about their current clinical performance. Mugford *et al.* (1991) and Palmer *et al.* (1995) believe that such an approach is likely to be effective where:

- the practitioners themselves have agreed to participate;
- feedback is timely and occurs quickly after the actual audit;
- the audit relates to an area over which the practitioner has some degree of control;
- there is a clear rationale about why the practice needs to change;
- the proposed change is manageable, or it can be broken down into smaller parts to make it manageable.

Marion's story (Box 2.4) provides us with a number of pieces of information about the use of audit to develop practice. It also highlights that the development of practice may not always mean changing the way in which the nurse practices. In this situation, the trigger to develop practice was the realization that the final night of each shift was much busier in terms of accidents. Marion and Claire were able to use this initial realization that something unusual was happening as the basis for an audit of accident reports. This audit provided the evidence, that the final shift was indeed busier with accidental injuries. However, the audit was not able to identify whether this was related to the duration of the shifts. Marion and Claire were able to convince the management that this might be the reason, and thus the factory moved from a three-shift system to a four-shift one. In order that Marion and Claire can prove the effectiveness of the change, they will need to continue to audit accident reports over the next few months to identify whether the new shift system has resulted in fewer accidental injuries. This example clearly demonstrates that sometimes the development of practice needs to occur when the evidence for change is less than optimum. Without changing the shift system, Marion and Claire would never know whether the system of working long night shifts had an impact on the rate of accidental injury.

Reflection

The notion of reflective practice in nursing has become increasingly prominent. While reflection both in and on practice has become a central component of many nurse education programmes, its usefulness as a form of evidence has been less well articulated. Boyd and Fales (1983: 99) define reflection as part of a learning process which involves 'internally examining and exploring an issue of concern, triggered by an experience, which creates and clarifies meaning in terms of self, and which results in changed conceptual perspective'.

Several authors (Mezirow 1981; Boyd and Fales 1983; Schön 1991) have identified stages in the reflective process. These can be grouped collectively in three categories: awareness, critical analysis and finally, the formulation of a new perspective.

- *Awareness* – this category involves the gradual realization that the current method of practice is less than optimum in dealing with a particular patient's problems or needs. This realization may occur for a number of reasons, including an awareness of another method of care delivery, or an awareness of new literature that supports changing practice.
- *Critical analysis* – this is a constructive phase where the practitioner analyses both feelings and knowledge. While this stage may involve an analysis of existing knowledge in the form of literature, it may also involve the generation of new knowledge about a more effective method of care delivery.
- *Formulation of a new perspective* – at this stage, the practitioner is able to make a decision about what, if anything, needs to change and how future care should be delivered.

From the three general stages it is possible to identify that within practice development reflection can be used in several ways. First, reflection can assist the practitioner to identify the need for development. This results from what is often referred to as the awareness stage in a reflective process (Boyd and Fales 1983). As highlighted earlier, this stage is triggered by an awareness of uncomfortable feelings and thoughts about unmet need, or the comprehension that there may be a more effective way of delivering a certain aspect of care.

Second, reflection can occur during the process of developing practice. Such reflection may be triggered by something that goes particularly well, or by something that does not go as planned. These critical incidents are a major source of evidence about the process of developing practice. Chell (1998) used critical incidents recording as part of a study examining the process of studying managerial innovation. She found that critical incident recording allowed her to study innovation in the context in which it was occurring, and thus participants were able to detail previously unanticipated events. Reflection upon the process of developing practice will not provide evidence that one aspect of care delivery is more effective than another. However it does provide much needed awareness of the best way to manage the introduction of a new way of working. This awareness may then become a central part of the knowledge needed for the more widespread introduction of a development across the organization.

Finally, formulating a new perspective may lead to the generation of knowledge about a better way of delivering an aspect of care. This type of evidence is widely used within health care as the basis for further development. While the notion of a 'good idea' as a source of evidence may be open to criticism from some quarters, it is useful to remember that without an initial good idea, or at least a 'hunch' that this might improve care, practice would never advance. The important point about the use of good ideas is that they must be subject to evaluation and further research to identify the benefits. Otherwise there is the risk that practitioners waste resources delivering ineffective and possibly harmful health care to patients.

Vera's story (Box 2.5) illustrates the value of reflection during and after the development of practice. After Vera and Claire had been involved in the development, they both reflected upon it, and how it was introduced during their supervision session. With hindsight, it would have been much more appropriate if they had considered the context in which the development was going to operate. This would have allowed them to identify the potential stakeholders who should have been involved in the initial discussions about the proposal. During the reflective process, Claire described how she felt that Dr Thornton's reactions had more to do with control than the fact that he was not the originator of the idea. She described that whenever Dr Thornton discussed the rapid response team, he always acknowledged that the idea had originally

Box 2.5   Vera's story

I had worked as a discharge liaison sister with the medical directorate for the last six years. Recently Claire, the respiratory nurse specialist, and I had started to engage in weekly clinical supervision sessions. Both Claire and I were actively involved in reducing the pressure on acute beds by facilitating early discharge of patients. However during one of our supervision sessions, Claire reflected upon how in many cases admission could be prevented if the level of support and care could be increased for patients at home with certain types of conditions, for example those with chronic pulmonary disease. Claire and I agreed that a rapid response team would go a long way towards reducing pressure on acute beds. Both Claire and I were regular attenders of the Primary Care Group (PCG) stakeholders' meeting, and we decided that this would be a useful forum for the presentation of our initial ideas. We presented our initial ideas to the group, and Eileen, the PCG manager, suggested that we arrange a meeting with her and the community manager to discuss a bid to the Health Improvement Programme (HImP) for the rapid response team. Over the next six weeks we worked together to develop a bid for a rapid response community nursing team. This was subsequently submitted to the HImP, and several months later Eileen rang Claire and me to inform us that the bid had been successful and to thank us both for our input.

Claire and I had little involvement from this point forward, because Anne, the community manager, took the lead role. Claire and I thought nothing more about it until two months later, when the advertisements for the first posts for the team were advertised. The day after the advertisements came out, Dr Thornton burst into my office and started shouting about how the community directorate was moving forward on a development related to respiratory care, without input from the medical directorate. Dr Thornton appeared very angry that he had not been consulted. I tried my best to calm him down, but he said that he was going to see the chief executive about this later that day. I felt that it would be inappropriate to tell him that Claire had been involved, and that the whole development had stemmed from our initial idea. Dr Thornton stormed out still muttering about community services taking over.

I quickly rang Claire to tell her of my encounter with Dr Thornton, and to warn her about how angry he was. Claire said that she would need to tell him about our involvement in the planning of the development before he found out by accident. She said that she would go and see him immediately, and she would let her directorate manager know as soon as possible.

Later that day, Claire rang to say that she had told Dr Thornton. She reported that he had gone totally ballistic at the news, that 'his' nurse had been involved in such a betrayal. Simon, the directorate manager, had taken a different view, praising both Claire's and my vision in suggesting the development. However, he did feel that we had been somewhat misguided in not discussing it within the directorate first. Claire said that she felt that Dr Thornton might never speak to her again, as he had been very angry to find out that I had sold out to the 'community lot'.

Over the next few weeks there was a great deal of political manoeuvring within the trust. Eventually Anne informed me that she had been asked by the chief executive to work closely with Dr Thornton with the planning of the rapid response team. The original adverts were withdrawn, and the posts redesigned and then readvertised. Eventually, the team came into existence. While the initial idea was the same as we had proposed, it was not managed in the way we had envisaged, as it was now an outreach team, managed by the medical directorate. This caused some problems with team working between the rapid response team and primary care, but despite these, the project did appear to be successful.

been developed by staff from his team. Clearly Dr Thornton was keen to ensure that he was able to retain control over the care of the patients who had previously been admitted under his care. However Claire did feel that the leadership of the rapid response team by a doctor was slightly misleading, as the medical care to the patients being cared for by the team was provided by the patients' general practitioners. Finally, both Vera and Claire felt that despite the fact that the development was working well, it needed to be systematically evaluated to ensure that it was reaching its original objectives of preventing admission to an acute bed. Some of the GPs felt that some of the patients being cared for by the team would not have been admitted in the past, but rather, they would have been cared for by their relatives and primary care staff.

◯ Some fundamental principles: now and the future

From our discussions, we can draw out a number of fundamental principles about practice development.

1 Development is part of good practice. It is not an activity that should be added onto a role, undertaken after the 'work' has finished or be regarded as 'not normal' practice by managers or colleagues. Similarly, it is not an activity that can be undertaken by someone from outside the environment of care delivery, although they may usefully act as a facilitator in examining concepts of care.

2 Development is about collaboration and mutual learning. Practice developments are not sustainable, if they are thought to be possible, only by 'special' people who are either particularly clever, obsessed or employed to do it. Developing practice must involve everyone, and is an activity in which everyone can learn. Furthermore, it is an activity that has no endpoint. As more is learned, so more is seen to need to be learned.

3 The primary aim is to change practice in a local environment. The work must therefore take place somewhere, or with an aspect of care, over which people have some control. The work is not primarily concerned with its applicability to other settings or traditional research criteria, such as 'generalizability' but rather, emphasizes its evolving nature, relevance to practice and transferability to other settings through articulation of the local contexts of care policy, delivery and receipt.

4 Practice development is about challenging and examining key concepts and values that inform practice, and reorientating ourselves to a view of health care that is led by service users, rather than services and organizations. It is not about perpetuating inherited aspects of professional practice. This is a theoretical aspect of the work of practice development which, for example, allows exploration of what is truly meant by 'better' practice. For whom are we improving practice, and what criteria do we use to evaluate a better practice?

In thinking about the impact that a development may have in the future, we may be justifiably anxious that all our hard work will be undone. Again, it is more helpful to think of practice development as a continually evolving process, rather than as a time-limited project that leaves the door open for practice to revert instead of continually moving forward. There are some key ways in which we can ensure that practice developments actually make an enduring difference to the care that service users receive (Balfour and Clarke 2001). Many of these you will recognize as being entirely consistent with the key messages of this chapter.

- Enhance practitioner ownership of the development through recognition of the knowledge base of the practitioners, as well as the research-based evidence. People will persist with something, even when it is difficult to do so, if they feel that it is something that belongs to them.
- Promote 'deep' professional change, in which people learn to think about the needs and care of service users in a different way. It is very hard to undo people's learning.
- Expose the philosophy behind the actions of practitioners. Understanding why something is done in a particular way helps them to be more critical practitioners, recognizing the strengths and limitations of different practice philosophies.
- Create whole organization or intersystem change in which the change causes more than its core focus to change. The more organizational and professional systems support a development, the more easily it will become a core and an accepted activity across the organization and within all professional groupings.

◯ Conclusion

We hope that this chapter has highlighted the complexity of identifying and using evidence when developing practice. The shift in health and social care towards embracing evidence-based practice that exclusively calls for practitioners to use empirically derived knowledge has left many practitioners feeling excluded and disenfranchised. We hope that this chapter has successfully argued that there is a time and a place for knowledge derived from practical experience, user perspectives, reflection and audit. An inclusive, rather than exclusive, approach to the use of evidence in practice will allow practitioners and academics to work in partnership. Both have an equally important role in developing practice, and by working together, the debate about the theory–practice gap might be finally laid to rest. As Griffiths (1999: 146) has stated,

> A systematic questioning approach . . . does not contradict intuitive decision making, rather it simply demands a more rigorous approach to what constitutes research based knowledge and demands more searching questions about the intuitive decisions once made.

This statement might be seen to be as relevant to developing practice as it is to decisions made for individual patient care. Practitioners need to gain confidence in using their 'grumbles' and gut feelings in identifying where practice might be developed. Research-based evidence may then be drawn upon to ascertain the type of intervention that should be used, or ascertain the known effectiveness of a proposed intervention. In the later stages of practice development, it is important to use evaluation as a further source of evidence. However we have noted that traditional evaluation techniques are rarely appropriate in practice development and to do evaluation well, practitioners need to be mindful of a number of factors, for example timescales and ethical issues.

Clearly, evidence to support the development of practice is often complex and multifaceted. For practitioners to be able to sell their ideas, and to see the process through successfully, they need to pay a great deal of attention to, and articulate the nature and source of the evidence upon which they have drawn. This is a knowledge base to which practitioners may be contributing themselves, since the developments of today are the knowledge of tomorrow.

Part (II) The process of developing practice

③ Managing the development of practice

John Unsworth

◯ Chapter summary

While the concept of practice development is nebulous and ill defined, most nurses can recognize when they and their colleagues are engaged in the process. Like research, writers often present the process of developing their practice as very linear. This can lead to practitioners becoming confused when their attempts to introduce change are met with barriers and resistance. This chapter explores the nature of practice development in nursing, describing how individual, organizational and structural factors can either drive or suppress it. The implementation of most developments in practice draws heavily upon the theories of introducing change and innovation. Indeed, within this chapter, the author asserts that practice development is merely a specialized form of innovation. Managing the development of practice, whether as a practitioner, manager or facilitator, is a complex process which involves considerable skill in balancing the needs and desires of patients, professionals and the organization. Indeed, it is these interpersonal aspects of practice development activity that often make the process seem messy and uncoordinated. By examining actual developments, we hope to illustrate how success can be achieved, and failure minimized. Finally, the 'laggards' get their day, when the chapter looks at the nature of resistance to change, and how and why people react as they do to proposed changes in their day to day work.

◯ Introduction

Practice development is now a key feature of modern health care delivery. Health care professionals are being encouraged to develop both their individual practice and the services which they provide. Such changes have been driven, in part, by the ever increasing drive towards efficiency and quality in the National Health Service. The development of practice is of prime importance to health care organizations; very simply, 'health care organisations face a stark choice, innovate and change, or expect to be replaced by organisations that do' (Manion 1993: 41). Practice development is already used as part of the health commissioning process, and indeed, as mentioned in Chapter 1, the proliferation of such activity owes much to the creation of the internal market in the NHS. The development of practice is often an eclectic mix of the actual development of clinical practice and other related concepts like professional development. This has resulted in problems with definition, which, in turn, make the measurement of practice development problematic. Joyce (1999) suggests that this confusion is partly a result of the use of the terms interchangeably, both in the literature and as part of job titles. Practice development has been used within various professions and contexts. Within nursing, it usually refers to the development of clinical work, while in other professions it can relate to the marketing of the business of a professional such as accountancy practice. The term is also widely used in relation to the research process, where it refers to either the implementation of research findings into practice or the use of participative research methods such as action research.

Within a professional bureaucracy like the NHS, professionals are expected to plan and introduce innovations into their own practice. This situation is very different to the planning of innovation in other businesses. A large manufacturing company is likely to have a specific department that has responsibility for the development of new products before they are introduced into the wider company. It could be argued that the NHS has attempted to implement a similar type of development department with the establishment of practice development directorates or the establishment of practice or nursing development units.

Not only is the concept of practice development nebulous and difficult to define, but the term is also used interchangeably with those of innovation and change. Indeed, as you will see, the terms are used interchangeably within this book. This leads us to ask whether there is, in fact, a difference between the terms change, innovation and practice development? No one would doubt that the process of developing nursing practice draws heavily upon innovation and change theory, and this may be partly responsible for the confusion around terminology. It is important to consider whether practice development is simply another way of describing innovation. Later in this chapter, we will examine how innovation differs from practice development. First, let us examine what practice development is.

Several authors have attempted to define practice development. McCormack *et al.* (1999: 256) worked with a group of practice development nurses to develop the following definition:

> Practice development is a continuous process of improvement towards increased effectiveness in person centred care, through the enabling of nurses and health care teams to transform the culture and context of care. It is enabled and supported by facilitators committed to a systematic, rigorous and continuous process of emancipatory change.

While this definition is interesting, in so much as it recognizes that practice development is a continuous and incremental process, it is also open to criticism. The main criticism surrounds the notion that practice development requires an identified facilitator. Many individual practitioners may plan, implement and evaluate changes in their own sphere of practice. Other attempts at definition have involved the identification of the critical attributes of practice development as a concept (Unsworth 2000). This analysis suggested that practice development in its purest form involves:

- the introduction of new ways of working, which leads to a direct measurable improvement in the care or service to a client;
- changes that occur as a response to a specific client need or problem;
- changes that lead to the development of effective services;
- the maintenance or expansion of the business or work of the professional or organization.

Box 3.1 illustrates these critical attributes within an example of practice development. The figure suggests that this is an example of practice

---

Box 3.1   An illustration of a practice development

A district nurse working in a busy practice is concerned about the way she and her colleagues are caring for patients with leg ulceration. One patient, Mrs Morse, has had ulceration for 12 years, and despite the nurses' best efforts, her ulcers show little signs of improving. The nurse is aware that good assessment and compression therapy, if the ulcer is venous, would lead to rapid improvement, but is unable to obtain a Doppler to record ankle brachial pressure index. The nurse discusses this issue with her manager, who agrees to fund the purchase of a Doppler. Once available, the nurse is able to assess Mrs Morse's leg ulcer and the underlying aetiology, and finds that the ulcer is indeed venous in origin. The nurse commences compression using a multilayer system and Mrs Morse's ulcer is healed within six weeks.

development, because it clearly demonstrates the defining attributes of the concept. The assessment and subsequent healing of Mrs Morse's ulcer is a direct and measurable improvement in the care of the client. In turn, this was clearly a response to a specific client need or problem, which ultimately produced a more effective service, because of the elevation of suffering to the client and a reduction in the nurse's work.

One of the key elements of Unsworth's (2000) definition, is the notion that practice development should always be patient focused. While many people might think that this goes without saying, not all developments allow for the measurement of clear patient outcomes. McCormack *et al.* (1999) believe that there has been a paradigm shift, in recent years, away from the early developments in the 1980s, which centred around professionalization, such as the nursing process, towards more humanistic development. The 1990s have been characterized by development, which places patient outcomes at the centre of activity. Such developments have been driven, in part, by the clinical effectiveness agenda; this was discussed in more detail in Chapter 2. Another element in this definition is that of the development of effective services. There are a number of ways in which such effectiveness can be judged. This may be the implementation of clinically effective practice, which leads to improvement in patient outcome, for example, maximized independence after hip replacement. However, effectiveness can also be judged using other criteria, such as cost or the best use of resources. Therefore a new health visitor-led sleep clinic may be judged as effective because it reduces the need for individual home visits and therefore allows for the better use of health visiting time.

Finally, from an organizational perspective, practice development should also lead to the maintenance or expansion of the business or work. This attribute suggests why practice development has grown in importance since the implementation of commissioning. NHS organizations with a track record of innovative services are more likely to attract more business and contracts from surrounding areas. However, the reforms of the NHS structure (DOH 1997a) mean that there is, theoretically, less competition between NHS Trusts, so this attribute may assume less importance in the future. The isolation of critical attributes is useful in providing measurable criteria for the development of practice. However, the use of methods of concept analysis, developed by Walker and Avant (1995), have been criticized because they remove the concept being studied from its context. Given that practice development is often combined with other related activity, such as professional development, to what extent developing a separate definition is useful, is open to question.

As described earlier, it is important to identify whether practice development is simply another way of describing innovation. The *Oxford English*

Dictionary (Oxford University Press 1992) defines innovation as 'to bring in novelties and make changes'. However, the idea that innovation is always a novelty has been refuted by Damanpour (1987) who believes that innovation is not necessarily new. One of the most widely used definitions of innovation is that provided by West and Farr (1990: 9):

> the intentional introduction and application within a role, group or organisation of ideas, processes, products or procedures, new to the relevant unit of adoption, designed to significantly benefit the individual, the group, organisation or society.

West and Farr (1990) describe how innovation always has the intentionality of benefit. As a result, the definition above describes a broad range of people or groups who may derive benefit from the innovation. However, in practice development the emphasis is on improvement. While these words are similar, benefit is defined as 'advantage', while improvement implies 'making better' (Oxford University Press 1992). Therefore practice development does not necessarily make the delivery of care or services more advantageous for the practitioner or society, but it should always be perceived as an improvement by the individual patient/client. An innovation, on the other hand, might be advantageous to both the practitioner and the patient/client. This is illustrated through King's (1989: 17) definition of innovation within a health care setting:

> innovation is the sequence of activities by which a new element is introduced into a social unit, with the intention of benefiting the unit, some part of it or the wider society. The element need not be entirely novel or unfamiliar to members of the unit, but it must involve some discernable change or challenge to the status quo.

These definitions suggest that innovation differs from practice development, as defined within this book, in several respects. Innovation is not necessarily a response to an identified patient/client need. Nor is it directly related to the development of effective services, although it could be argued that an innovation that is of benefit to the group or organization should relate to effectiveness. Despite these subtle differences, there are several similarities. These include the fact that both innovation and practice development are a planned process that has a clear social and applied component, which means that they impact directly upon others. Given the suitable differences, it could be assumed that practice development is simply a specialized form of innovation, which occurs within a professional bureaucracy.

◯ Factors that influence development

There are literally hundreds of factors that can have either a positive or negative effect on the development of practice. In this section, the major factors that affect community nursing practice will be discussed. It is vitally important that practitioners or change facilitators are aware of many of these factors, so they are able to harness the positive influences to drive change forward, while at the same time avoiding some of the hazards associated with the negative factors. The factors can be divided into those that are related to the context in which the practice is to be developed, those that relate to the organization's structure, and those that relate to the influence of individuals within the organization.

Contextual factors

Chapter 1 examined several contextual variables in depth, and this high-lighted that policy can have a major impact on development at a local level. While some of this policy may be rigid and sometimes restrictive, because it is very prescriptive about how something should be implemented, other policies allow for local adaptation or interpretation. While the national agenda can provide stimulus for development and is often accompanied by resources, it can create conflict for managers and practitioners, because of the tensions between the 'must dos' from policy and the 'would like to dos' from practitioners. This suggests that the local agenda takes second place to the national agenda on many occasions. Recently the national agenda has been so large, it is likely that many local projects have been shelved because of problems related to the capacity within the service for development. As well as national and local agendas, contextual factors such as seasonal variations in demand and waiting lists can also have an impact. For community nurses these changes mean that patients, who might have previously been cared for in hospital, are now cared for at home or within intermediate care facilities. Additionally, patients are discharged sooner and therefore have greater nursing needs when they get home. These factors can have a negative effect on development, because they reduce the capacity for the planning and delivery of new services. On the other hand, they can also provide the impetus for the development of innovative ways of delivering care, such as winter pressure units and nurse-led beds (Unsworth *et al.* 2000).

Structural and organizational

The structure of the organization and its culture can make or break an idea, and its influence is widespread and often misread. Manion (1993) suggests that successful organizations have established an internal climate that supports entrepreneurial activity. Such an environment needs to go beyond the paying of lip service to the ideas of innovation and employee development. One of the key positive indicators of an innovative organization is its size (Kimberly and Evanisko 1981). In this case, size is important because the bigger the organization in terms of beds, manpower or budget, the more development will occur within that organization. Obviously, large organizations will have greater amounts of development just by virtue of their size. However, large organizations also have a number of advantages over their smaller counterparts, as these organizations often cover large geographical areas and have less competition from surrounding NHS Trusts. Many larger organizations also have more organizational resources, both human and financial, to devote to the development of practice. Damanpour (1987) refers to this capacity as organizational slack, and suggests that the additional resources such slack can provide have a positive effect on the adoption of technological innovations, which may demand considerable investment. Similarly, organizations which are highly specialized are likely to be more successful at encouraging development (Kimberly and Evanisko 1981). Peters and Waterman (1982), in their study of America's most successful companies, suggested that a key feature of a successful organization was that it concentrated on its strengths. Highly specialized teams, or NHS Trusts, are therefore more likely to be successful in terms of developing practice if they concentrate on areas that they already do well. One of the problems of the creation of the internal market in health care was the diversification that occurred in an attempt to capture new business from other NHS organizations. This situation created duplication of services and wasted already scarce NHS resources.

Within the NHS, many health care providers are divided into structured divisions or directorates. Such divisions can have both a positive and negative effect on the development of practice. First, divisions allow for devolved decision making, and it is probably easier therefore to get support or permission for a proposed development. However, divisions can make the implementation of corporate development throughout the organization more complex. Another feature of divisions within an organization is that it creates a strong sense of identity for its members. This can facilitate development by strengthening ownership and creating healthy competition between departments. Kimberly and Evanisko (1981) refer to the subdivision of health organizations as functional differentiation; they suggest that such differentiation can cause problems with the implementation of whole organization innovation, but is helpful when introducing very specific measures that affect one or two departments.

The organization's view of risk and risk management can also influence how practitioners and managers are able to develop practice. Many organizations seek to implement universal developments in practice across the organization as a risk reduction or management strategy. Such development, like the implementation of pressure sore risk assessment tools, while laudable, can cause problems, because no one tool is ideal for every clinical setting. As a result, stafff are forced to use a tool that overpredicts risk in their clinical setting. Essentially, universal developments are rarely ideal, and what organizations should be seeking is what Peters and Waterman (1982) describe as simultaneous centralization and decentralization. In this situation, the organization would indicate that all clinical areas need a pressure sore risk assessment tool. However each ward and department would be able to select the best tool for their own clinical setting. Kramer (1990: 35) stresses that 'success comes from allowing each team to do its own thing, because each team is unique and works in unique circumstances'. Managers and practitioners need to be concerned with one thing when operating in a culture that encourages corporate decision making with local implementation, that is, each group of staff do the right thing for the right reasons. The flexibility afforded by local implementation would make it all too easy to ignore the need for practice to be continually reviewed and developed.

Another major factor for the NHS which can have a positive effect on the development of practice is how stable the management structure is. Many NHS organizations are currently, or have recently been, restructured either because of local changes or as a result of changes in national policy, for example the creation of Primary Care Trusts. Such changes serve to destabilize innovation in practice for several reasons. Sometimes it is difficult to gain permission for a proposed change, because managers are new or because the existing managers are fearful of rocking the boat in case they fail to get their own or another management position. Instability in the management structure also affects practitioners, making them less likely to want to work on a new project or change the way they work. This is especially so if a new manager has been appointed, because staff are treading carefully before wanting to propose radical change or different ways of working. Instability in management structures can also drive the need for rapid visible change within the clinical setting. Managers may have a short time period to prove they are capable of doing their job, and may encourage practitioners to develop their practice and clinical services quickly. Sometimes these services and changes are very successful. However, the rapid development of such services can reduce the sustainability of the new way of working, and as a result, the change only exists while the manager is in post.

Another issue about the modern management of health care within the NHS, is that managers often have responsibility for the management of more than nursing services. This can have a positive effect, because it allows for the establishment of patient-focused and multidisciplinary developments around specific conditions or clinical problems. However, the down side is that it can result in the management resources being spread very thinly. This in turn, reduces the amount of time a manager is able to devote to directly supporting individual projects. Within primary care, this is further compounded by the fact that services can be geographically spread, and this can lead to practitioners feeling increasingly isolated. These could be some of the reasons why new posts around the facilitation of practice development, that is practice development nurses, have been established by some NHS Trusts.

One of the main negative factors to influence the development of practice is resources. In the past the NHS has been guilty of concentrating too much on financial management. The development of practice may initially be resource intensive and require capital or revenue funding for training, equipment purchase or the establishment of new posts. It may take many years to realize the savings from these changes, if indeed it is possible to realize savings at all. Many developments save staff time, but the money from this often cannot be released, as the staff are still in post after the development has been introduced. Obviously, these staff can use their time in new ways, such as developing their public health role, but the developments still require additional funding. The introduction of Corporate and Clinical Governance may add new impetus to develop practice, by freeing up NHS organizations from being judged purely on financial terms. As a result, developments in practice which improve patient outcomes and the quality of service provision will also be measured as part of the way in which NHS Trust performance is judged.

Finally, organizational factors such as centralized decision making and formalization, that is the need to seek approval for a development, can have a negative effect on the development of practice. However, managers may argue that it is essential for them to know what is going on in their own patches, so that legal issues and risk assessment can be formally undertaken. However, there is a difference between keeping people informed, and seeking formal permission to develop clinical practice. Essentially, if decision making is devolved, it should be possible to gain permission for any development, either from the practitioner's line manager or the next manager above them, without needing to seek approval from a whole myriad of individuals.

Individual factors

There are numerous factors related to both practitioners and managers, which can positively or negatively affect the development of practice. Some of the most influential of these factors will be discussed here, while others related to people's reactions of change are discussed later in this chapter.

One of the most influential of all individual factors is the empowerment of practitioners to develop. While empowerment is a key part of what encourages practitioners to initiate or adopt developments, it is not the whole story. Not all practitioners who are empowered will initiate developments in their practice, and, even those who do may still experience problems negotiating their way around the implementation of developments that cross professional groups or the primary/secondary care interface. Manion (1993: 41) believes that 'effective innovations are developed by individuals who know the organisation at its core'. Perhaps this is the key to why some practitioners are able to initiate and implement developments in practice while others experience problems. Characteristically, practitioners who lead the development of practice have been in an organization for at least a 10-year period (Clarke *et al.* 1998). This has important implications for the educational preparation of specialist practitioners, which sometimes involves them initiating a development in practice. This is discussed in depth in Chapter 5. Clearly this suggests that clinical areas with rapid staff turnover or unstable workforces are unlikely to be able to develop sustainable changes in practice.

Mason *et al.* (1991: 5) states that 'health care institutions are highly complex organisations, where change does not come easily. Many nurses have been frustrated in their attempts to bring about change that would improve and facilitate their everyday practice'. There appears to be an assumption within some parts of the NHS that the new management cultures will automatically encourage practitioners to develop their own practice. Many people are surprised when practitioners fail to take advantage of their newfound freedom from previously tight management control. Mason *et al.* (1991: 5) states that 'it cannot be assumed that nurses have the confidence or skills to make changes in their workplace in politically astute ways'.

Given the problems that practitioners may experience in initiating developments in practice, any assistance they can get from either a facilitator or a manager will be helpful. One way in which managers or other senior clinicians may help is to act as a product champion. This is a person who has the ability to provide both practical support and negotiate with senior managers within the organization to smooth the introduction of the proposed development. Cauthorne-Lindstrom and Tracy (1992) describe how product champions are key individuals who are not necessarily in positions of power but who have the unquestionable backing of senior executives. Champions are used to generate enthusiasm, work the system to secure resources, and provide people with information about the progress of the development. The development of practice can also be facilitated by the individual manager's management style. Styles that are open, supportive and based upon mutual trust can give confidence to practitioners to take forward ideas and initiatives. Equally important are the interpersonal relationships with the individual primary health care team. West and Wallace (1991) found that innovative teams in primary care had peer leadership, team cohesiveness and a positive team climate.

⭕ Using change theories in the development of practice

Lancaster (1999) describes several types of change, including developmental, haphazard and spontaneous. Most types of change can be divided into two broad categories: planned and unplanned. Planned change involves the intentional and deliberate introduction of a new idea. As its name suggests, planned change involves the process of planning, and the introduction of the new idea into the work environment should ideally be well thought out. Unplanned change on the other hand, is the introduction of a new idea or way of working without any preparation. This can be either haphazard change or spontaneous, that is a reaction to an event. Both categories of change can be either introduced by management or the organization (top-down) or identified, planned and implemented by practitioners (bottom-up).

Carson (1999) describes how there are numerous theories of planned change, but all of these involve four key stages. These stages are the recognition of either the innovation or the unmet need, implementation of the innovation, consolidation and finally evaluation. An understanding of change theories can be useful to practitioners seeking to implement changes in their practice because they provide a framework for the planning and implementation of the new development. In this section, a summary of the major points of three change theories will be presented, together with a discussion related to the practical application of each theory to nursing practice.

Kurt Lewin's field theory

The development of classical change theory is accredited to Lewin (1951) who developed field theory, which is essentially a way of describing a here and now situation, in which an individual participates (De Rivera 1976). The notion of field theory in relation to change is important, because as the field or situation changes, the change agent will need to alter his or her approach accordingly. As such, the field is not static, but changes over time, and is influenced by internal and external forces. These influences, which consist of both driving and restraining forces, can be considered as a force field. In situations where the driving forces are greater than the restraining forces, change can be implemented.

Lewin (1951) described how individuals introducing change need to undertake a careful estimation of the strength of the influences for and against the proposed development.

Another major part of field theory was the examination of individual – group relationships. Lewin (1958) postulated that groups don't make conscious decisions about the aims of the group, rather individuals within the group make decisions after a group discussion. Therefore it is possible to gain approval for a proposed change by influencing a number of key individuals within a group. Many practitioners who have introduced change into community or practice teams will have already realized that discussions with key individuals prior to a large group presentation can smooth the introduction of a new way of working. Similarly, if presenting to a group of managers, it is often useful to discuss your proposal with one or two members of the group. This will enable people to champion your cause during the meeting and subsequent discussion. Lewin (1951) described how ideas about change travel in channels through a social system. These ideas do not automatically enter or move through channels by themselves, and often they need someone to drive them forward. Within any social system or organization there are points of entry for new ideas. Gatekeepers such as team leaders and managers usually control these entry points. The rate at which communication about a new idea travels through a social system can be influenced by these gatekeepers, who can speed up or impede the progress of a new idea.

Lewin also described a sequence of strategies designed to bring about change. In any change process, permanency is the objective, although, in some cases, contextual and organizational factors act against this, for example short-term funding. The first phase in the change process involves a shaking up of the status quo, which Lewin described as unfreezing. Unfreezing involves increasing the motivation of the participants in preparation for the change. This stage also involves identifying and articulating the need for change. Lancaster and Lancaster (1983) identify that credibility and mutual trust are essential characteristics for the change agent during this part of the process. In the second stage, 'moving to a new level', involves the participants accepting the need for change, and collaborating to produce an action plan for the implementation of the new way of working. The final stage, 'refreezing', involves the new way of working being integrated into the participant's culture and pattern of working.

Everett Rogers' diffusion theory

Bushy (1992) described how Rogers' work expanded upon the previous work of Lewin. Rogers' work focused upon diffusion (dissemination)

Table 3.1   Summary of the stages of Rogers' diffusion model

Stage	Description
Knowledge	Awareness of an innovation's existence and understanding how it functions
Persuasion	Formulation of a favourable or unfavourable attitude towards the innovation
Decision	Deciding whether to adopt or reject the innovation
Implementation	Putting the innovation into use
Confirmation	Decision to continue or reject the new way of working

Table 3.2   Types of knowledge related to innovation adoption

Type of knowledge	Description
Awareness knowledge	What is it?
	How does it work?
How-to knowledge	How should it be used?
Principles knowledge	What are the underlying principles about how the innovation works?

and adoption (acceptance) of innovations. He described how individuals do not make an instantaneous decision about an innovation, but rather, decisions are made over a period of time. He described five stages to the process of decision making about an innovation or idea. Each of these stages is sequential in nature, but it is not uncommon to find that some of the stages overlap. Table 3.1 provides a summary of each of the stages.

Knowledge stage
This stage involves an individual becoming aware of the existence of an innovation or new way or working, and understanding how the innovation works in practice. Becoming aware of an innovation can happen in a number of different ways. The individual may be an information seeker and use peers or established networks to identify innovations in the areas of expertise. Similarly, an individual's own interests, needs and existing attitudes have a bearing upon both information seeking and subsequent adoption. Rogers referred to this as selective exposure. Finally, perception of a need for change is another important bearing upon whether an individual will be receptive to communication. Rogers (1995) described three types of knowledge (Table 3.2). Of these, change agents tend to concentrate on awareness knowledge, but greater emphasis

needs to be placed upon 'how-to knowledge' because this is the essential information that practitioners need to be able to try out the innovation, before full adoption.

Persuasion stage
The persuasion stage is concerned with the formulation of feelings and attitudes towards an innovation. Selective perception, which is a tendency to interpret messages in relation to existing beliefs, is important at this stage. The individual's perception of an innovation can be shaped by the characteristics that the innovation possesses. Rogers and Shoemaker (1971) have identified five essential characteristics a change should have if it is to be successful:

1 *Relative advantage* – This is the degree to which the new idea is considered superior to the old way of doing things.
2 *Compatibility* – How different is the new way of doing things? Major changes may need to be introduced slowly, because of the need to change behaviour, attitudes and organizational culture. To assist in the formulation of an attitude towards an innovation the individual may mentally apply the new idea to his or her own particular situation.
3 *Complexity* – How difficult is the new way of doing things? Refusal to adopt the new way of working may be a way of avoiding admitting that we don't understand.
4 *Trialability* – Can the idea be tried out on a small scale? Trialing an idea often demonstrates its usefulness to participants.
5 *Observability* – Can we tell if anything has changed?

Even after favourable feelings, or an attitude to the new idea has been formulated, adoption of the innovation does not automatically follow. Adoption at this stage can be assisted by contact with a near peer who is satisfied, having previously adopted the innovation. This is particularly useful when a change agent is encouraging adoption of an innovation across an organization, as staff involved in the initial pilot can be used to encourage colleagues to adopt the new idea or way of working.

Decision stage
This stage involves activities that lead an individual to either adopt or reject the proposed innovation. The decision stage may be characterized by anxiety about the potential consequences of the change. There are a number of ways of reducing this anxiety, including the use of small scale trials and demonstration sites. Individuals involved in these trials or demonstrations can be very effective at encouraging adoption, especially if they are credible, respected or leaders. It is important to remember that rejection of the new idea is also possible at this stage. Essentially, there are two types of rejection: active, which involves the individual

considering and even trialing the idea before rejecting it; and passive rejection, which involves either not really considering the idea, or simply forgetting about the initial communication of the idea.

Implementation stage
The implementation stage involves putting the idea, or new way of working, into use. It is at this stage that previously unforeseen problems can occur, and the change agent plays a pivotal role in troubleshooting and providing technical assistance. The implementation stage can continue for a long period of time, but eventually the aim is for the innovation to become accepted as part of the individual's everyday work. Rogers (1995) describes how reinvention can occur during implementation. This is where the individual changes the original innovation to fit their own circumstances. Whether this reinvention is considered good or bad depends upon the individual's viewpoint. From the perspective of the adopter, reinvention is beneficial because it can reduce the complexity of the innovation and increase compatibility with current practice. However organizations are often reluctant to allow reinvention, because it can cause problems with outcome measurement and evaluation.

Confirmation stage
During the confirmation stage, an individual seeks reinforcement about the decision made. This can be either reinforcement that the decision to adopt it was right, and it subsequently produced the right outcomes, or that the decision to reject the innovation was right. If the individual is uncomfortable about the decision that he or she made, they will be motivated to do something about it. It is possible at this stage for a person who had adopted the innovation to decide to abandon or significantly alter it, or alternatively a person who had previously rejected an innovation to decide to adopt it after all.

Gordon L. Lippitt's model of change

Lippitt's theory of change (Lippitt 1973) is formulated around the facilitation of change within an organization by an external change agent. He presents a seven stage process to change introduction.

Stage 1: Diagnosis of the problem
The first stage of the change process should involve the identification of the problem or unmet need that is to be addressed. The process of problem identification should involve the systematic collection and analysis of data, rather than be based solely on a hunch. During this stage, it is helpful if the change agent is able to encourage discussion and invite suggestions on the way forward from the people who will be affected by

the subsequent change. Similarly, early identification of the key stake-holders and the commencement of a dialogue with them will assist with the implementation of the change.

Stage 2: Assessment of motivation and capacity for change
This stage involves both the assessment of the people involved in the proposed change and the environment. The aim is to identify resources, constraints, change supporters and potential facilitators. Using the information gained from the assessment, the change agent should be able to draw up a list of possible solutions to the problem, and appraise the available options. While an assessment of motivation and capacity for change is an important stage, it is often poorly managed in the health service. Changes are often introduced with little regard for either workload or physical resources, such as space. Clarke (1997) describes how nurses are often required to develop their practice while at the same time continue to deliver the services they have always provided. There appears to be little understanding about the capacity of teams to develop, and many teams are encouraged to continue with innovations, rather than consolidate already established developments.

Stage 3: Assessment of change agent's motivation and capacity for change
During this stage, the organization would need to consider the appointed external change agent's credibility with the workforce. This may include an analysis of the strengths and weaknesses of the implementation team. Ideally, it is important to ensure that the implementation team have shared objectives and goals, and that they are 'singing from the same song sheet' and giving out consistent messages.

Stage 4: Selection of progressive change objectives
This is the planning stage, and as such, it involves the identification of a step by step plan for the implementation of the change. At the same time, the change agent may allocate tasks or areas of responsibility to key individuals, as well as identifying deadlines for the completion of each stage of the plan.

Stage 5: Choosing the appropriate role for the change agent
Lippitt identifies three roles that the change agent could adopt. These are expert role model, catalyst teacher and group leader. A change agent who is experienced in the field in which the change is being made may be able to take on an expert role. However, if the change agent is external to the organization, he or she would need to be widely recognized as an expert or leader in the field to maintain credibility within the organization. A catalyst teacher role would involve the change agent working to

keep the change on track, and would utilize the experience, skills and knowledge of the participants. Finally, a group leader role could be used if the proposed change had an identified steering group which had been charged with leading the change. The use of such a group is common when introducing large scale or organizational change. Whatever role the change agent has, it is important that both managers and the participants in the change, have similar expectations of that person.

Stage 6: Maintenance of the change
Once the change has been implemented, interest and enthusiasm may wane and practitioners may lapse into their old behaviour, thus affecting the sustainability of the new way of working or idea. The change agent can encourage continued participation by having regular contact and discussion with the participants.

Stage 7: Termination of the helping relationship
Finally, the change agent gradually withdraws from the organization or moves on to another project. It is important that ongoing responsibilities related to the monitoring and maintenance of the change are handed over to other people to ensure the sustainability of the change.

Problems with change theories

While change theories and models provide a useful framework for a change agent or practitioner to plan and introduce a new way of working, they all have a number of limitations. Most of the models are linear and are presented as unidirectional. This can lead to confusion when dealing with change in real life, as this is often a messy process, and can involve moving between stages in more than one direction, as contextual and organizational factors alter the original idea. Additionally, not all changes involve all of the stages in the exact order in which the models place them. This is especially the case where a practitioner is introducing a change from the grass roots. A great deal of planning may go into this change before the practitioner seeks the approval of the organization or starts to sell the idea to other colleagues.

Some models concentrate on the implementation of change by an organization, for example, Rogers' diffusion model, where others deal with the planning and implementation by individuals. However, one of the strengths of Rogers' model is that it can deal with the uncertainty presented by individuals who choose to adapt the innovation before adopting it. Other models assume that individuals within the organization have little or no impact on the implementation of a planned change.

⃝ Change strategies

Haffer (1986) describes three major categories of change strategy: empirical–rational, power–coercive and normative re-educative.

Empirical–rational strategy

This strategy is based upon the assumption that people will adopt change if it can be rationally justified, or if it is based upon scientific (empirical) evidence. When used in isolation, this strategy does not usually produce lasting change, because people often do not act rationally. One of the problems is that other factors can influence our decisions about whether to change, for example peer pressure, potential gain from the new way of working and the length of time the old behaviour had been practiced.

Power–coercive

This strategy is based upon the assumption that people will comply with the instructions of those people with greater power. Change using this strategy is usually top-down and, while the introduction of the change may be successful, the new way of working is dependent on the person with the power reinforcing the new way of working. Often once the person moves away or stops concentrating on that area of practice, the practitioners revert to their old behaviour. This strategy has in the past been widely used within the NHS partly as a response to the need for rapid visible change.

Normative re-educative

While the other two strategies are non-participative, participation is central to change introduced using a normative re-educative strategy. The practitioner is encouraged to be involved in planning, implementing and evaluating the change, and thus a more lasting change in practice is achieved. Using this strategy, the new way of working is integrated into the participant's value system.

While each of the change strategies may be used in isolation to introduce a development, they may also be used together over a period of time. This is illustrated by Emma's story (Box 3.2). Emma attempted to improve patient care by providing evidence of the need for change and appealing to practitioners that comprehensive assessment is a rational way of managing leg ulcers. This strategy had some initial success, with some practitioners complying with the new way of working. Later, concern that despite her best efforts the situation for some patients was unchanged, led Emma to use a power coercive strategy. This was achieved

Box 3.2   Emma's story: using different change strategies to implement a development

Emma Newby is an experienced tissue viability nurse working in a large community trust. Since she came into post two years ago, she has become increasingly concerned about the assessment of patients with leg ulceration. Together with the clinical audit group, Emma undertakes an audit to examine current practice. This reveals that very few patients have had a comprehensive assessment, and many have not had their ulcer diagnosed. She is very concerned that some patients are having compression bandages applied, even though the district nurses don't know, for certain, the type of ulcer. Working with a small multidisciplinary group of practitioners, she develops an assessment tool and sets about teaching nurses how to measure the patient's ankle brachial pressure index (ABPI) and how to apply compression bandages properly. Emma finds that the staff are very enthusiastic and attendance at the initial training is very good. The staff appear to be using the new assessment tool, and the trust purchases a number of Dopplers for use by staff.

One year later, Emma becomes concerned again, because of several instances when she is asked by general practitioners to assess patients. She again finds that many of the patients have not had their ABPIs measured, and time and time again, she is finding patients with poorly applied bandages. Emma is becoming increasingly frustrated that, although she is continually running training, attendance is very poor, and she has had to cancel several training sessions. Emma raises her concerns with managers and asks for suggestions. The managers feel that the issue is so important in terms of clinical risk that attendance at training will be made compulsory. Emma agrees to repeat the audit and produces league tables of compliance for the completion of assessment. These league tables are sent to all staff, and effectively set one general practice against another, in terms of the quality of their care. This new approach is very effective at ensuring staff are trained, and compliance with assessment of patients with leg ulceration improves. Three months later Emma repeats the audit and finds that all but a few patients have been assessed.

Eventually, all staff have attended training. Despite all staff being trained, there are still issues around competence to practice, and Emma is still coming across patients with poorly applied bandages. Emma works on a new approach, where each primary care group has a trainer who is responsible for identifying problems and providing regular updates for staff. Emma offers support to the trainers, who are able to audit colleagues' patient care, and identify problems as part of the clinical governance infrastructure.

Table 3.3   Assessing the potential for resistance during the introduction of change

---

- How great is the change?
- How reasonable is the change?
- How much are participants emotionally invested in the old way of working?
- How threatening to the participants is the new way of working?
  - Will it alter their role and power?
  - Will it alter the content of their job?
  - Will it alter the person's freedom to perform their job?
- How do participants feel about the change agent?
- How clear are people about what is expected of them?

---

through the use of league tables, effectively naming and shaming those practitioners who were failing to comply, and by making training compulsory for all staff. Finally, while all staff were compliant with the new way of working, there was still wide variation in the competence of practitioners. To improve this, a longer term normative re-educative strategy was used, with the provision of continued updating, regular feedback and the offer of continued support within the practice setting.

◯ Resistance to change

Resistance to any change or development in practice is a common occurrence. Change is rarely universally accepted by all staff working within a particular area. Essentially, resistance occurs for one of two reasons, either because a person does not like the proposed change, or because they have misconceptions about what the change will mean and how it will effect them. Lancaster (1999) reports that resistance reveals the human side of change, and it is often accompanied by feelings of fear, doubt and uncertainty. For whatever reason, people resist the proposed change. They rarely, if ever, resist simply because they wish to be obstructive or difficult. Change usually challenges the status quo, and can even seek to alter the values and beliefs of an individual work group; where this is the case resistance is likely to be high. King and Anderson (1995: 169) describe how 'those who stand to lose most, whether in terms of positional power, organisational resources, social contact at work or rewards, are likely to resist most vociferously'. Within the NHS, change often means an increased workload for those involved in it, and this is a common reason for resistance towards it (West and Anderson 1992).

Given the potential for resistance to proposed change, how can practitioners seeking to develop practice identify the types of resistance that may occur and what can they do to overcome or prevent this? Lancaster

---

Box 3.3   Vignette

Abbey Medical Group is a large general practice serving 14,000 patients in a large inner-city area. The newly integrated team is keen to identify a practice development on which the whole team can work. The team approaches Lynn, the practice development nurse, to ask her to help the team identify potential developments. During the process of identifying developments, the team identifies the need to improve bereavement care within the practice. The basis of this development is that, over the last few years, there have been a number of traumatic deaths affecting patients from the practice. Staff have often felt ill prepared to offer support and advice to relatives, and there is general agreement that this aspect of practice could be improved. Over the next few weeks, the team work with the clinical psychologist attached to the practice, to develop a system whereby all bereaved relatives would be offered a support visit eight weeks after the death of their loved one. Where patients refuse, they would be sent information on other types of support available, including voluntary groups. The planned programme also includes referral by the nursing team to the psychologist, if they identify that the patient is having an abnormal bereavement reaction. Staff also undergo an intensive training course to help them deal with bereavement and to assist them with assessment.

(1999) describes how it is possible to assess the potential degree of resistance. Some of the suggested assessment criteria are outlined in Table 3.3. Once the possible reasons for resistance have been identified, it should be possible to plan to defuse at least some of the resistance.

One crucial area is the notion of selling the idea. The way in which a change agent or practitioner sells the idea will differ in relation to both the nature and scope of the change and to whom the idea is to be sold. Box 3.3 highlights a development within one large general practice. This development was sold to the practitioner as an improvement in patient care and a new and exciting role for the nursing team. Essentially, its introduction was based around an empirical rational strategy, as the idea had a research basis and appeared very rational to the staff involved. Resistance to the development was high from some quarters because of the degree of additional work the proposed development would present. However it appeared that the individual practitioners, although unhappy about the proposal, went ahead with the majority decision in this case, and did not raise their dissent within the group meeting. The same idea was sold by the change agent to the NHS Trust, on the grounds that this would be a significant new innovation, which would attract interest in the organization's work from outside agencies. So essentially, the idea was sold in an altruistic way to practitioners, and as a way of increasing the organization's kudos to the NHS Trust. The issue of kudos is interesting as it allows practitioners to sell developments to an organization, which require additional resources or may even carry considerable risk.

Another important factor in overcoming resistance is encouraging ownership and involvement. If the people affected by the proposed change feel that they can adapt the change slightly during its implementation, they are less likely to resist it than if they are presented with a change that is a fait accompli. In order to encourage ownership, the person proposing change must ensure that the exact details of the change, including how it is likely to affect the practitioners, must be communicated effectively. This can often prove problematic, because the preparatory work may lead to leaks about what is proposed. Such leaks can result in resistance, because of misconceptions about how the proposed change will affect people. Similar problems can occur as a result of the appointment of a change agent, such as a practice development nurse, where different practitioners will have different misconceptions about their role. One way round this problem is to involve opinion leaders in the initial planning of the change. Opinion leaders are well respected practitioners who will be able to influence the views of other individuals over a period of time and thereby reduce resistance to the development.

Another way of looking at resistance is to consider the characteristics of the people you are expecting to adopt the proposed development. Rogers (1995) outlines five categories of adopters to describe why people don't all adopt an innovation at the same time. These five categories represent ideal types, and it is possible to find exceptions to these groupings. Additionally, individuals may display different characteristics depending upon the type of change proposed. So a practitioner with an interest in wound care may be an early adopter of a development related to wound care, but may be a laggard when faced with a new method of continence assessment.

- *Innovators* – These account for 2.5 per cent of people. These people are likely to be outside the local circle and tend to form friendships with other innovators. To be an innovator, a person requires access to resources and the ability to understand and apply complex knowledge to a practical situation.
- *Early adopters* – These account for 13.5 per cent of people. Early adopters are an integral part of any social system, because they tend to be opinion leaders from whom others seek advice and information.
- *Early majority* – These account for 34 per cent of people. This group of people adopt a new idea just before the others. As a group, they rarely, if ever, lead and may deliberate for some time before they decide to adopt the new way of working.

- *Late majority* – These account for 34 per cent of people. This group adopt the new way of working just after the early majority. It is likely that adoption occurs simply because of the increasing pressure from peers who have already adopted.
- *Laggards* – These account for 16 per cent of people. This group are the last people to adopt the new way of working. They often refer to past failures as a reason for not adopting, such as 'we tried it before and it didn't work'.

An alternative way of looking at why people adopt a new way of working more quickly than others is to consider the notion of team roles (Belbin 1993). This work identifies a number of specific team roles which people may have within an organization. Several roles are identified, including *resource investigators* who are seen as popular team members, able to identify potential developments in practice by contacting others outside of the organization already working on a similar project. Resource investigators rarely initiate a new development, but instead rely upon others to drive the development forward. *Plants*, on the other hand, are often the source of ideas and proposals. Plants are intellectual and imaginative, but at the same time they rarely pay attention to details and can become bored with an idea before it is fully implemented. Plants work well with *completer finishers*, who are able to make sure deadlines are met and that details are checked. Another major role is that of *team worker*. The team worker is dependable and ensures that the work gets done. They effectively hold the team together during periods of change.

Using Belbin's team roles enables people to think differently about the development of practice. Practitioners who are *plant shapers*, who lead to initiation of new ideas, are only able to do so because other people are ensuring that the day to day work of the organization is completed. Thinking in this way means that everyone has a role to play in the development of practice, even if they do not take an active role in its introduction.

◯ Conclusion

This chapter has explored the process of developing practice, looking particularly at models that assist with the process of introducing planned change. Clearly, practice development is a complex process which requires considerable skill to manage. While models of change are useful in some cases, they often oversimplify the introduction of any development. Within the chapter, the impact of organizational, structural and individual factors has been described. Many of these factors act as antecedents, driving forward the development of practice. However, it is important to realize that these factors may also influence development during its introduction. Being aware of such influences is an important part of managing any development.

Another key skill which the practitioner introducing a development requires, is the ability to identify and plan how to deal with resistance to change. Many developments hit problems because of an inability to successfully deal with interpersonal aspects of the development of practice.

4) Concepts of risk in the development of practice

Glenda Cook and Wilma W. Ayris

◯ Chapter summary

This chapter will explore influences on the ways in which practitioners identify and manage uncertainty and risk in their efforts to develop their practice. It is recognized that risk is implicit in many aspects of practice, particularly in situations where practice is changed and developed. Such situations may place the individual practitioner and their employing organization in a tenuous position. Therefore strategies for moving practice forward within current health and social care policy as well as legal and professional practice frameworks will be discussed to promote innovation in practice, while actively seeking to manage risk. The chapter will start by examining the nature of risk in health care, and then move on to explore the assessment and management of risk in practice development.

◯ Introduction

Meeting the needs of the service user is a central concern to all practitioners, regardless of the level within the infrastructure in which the individual practises. Service commissioners/planners, managers and those involved in direct contact with clients face the challenge of responding to client needs. The ways in which these challenges are addressed differ, reflecting their individual practice perspective and the scope or limitation of their decision making capacity. Inevitably, this leads to conflict and frustration between responding to the needs of the individual client and/or community and working within the constraints of the organization. Practitioners who strive toward enhancing the quality of services through developing new and innovative practices, face the challenge of managing the uncertainties inherent in new developments, including identification and management of risks to the client, practitioner and the organization. Although this may place the practitioner in a vulnerable position, such efforts are rewarded through the development of responsive client centred practice.

The purpose of this chapter is to explore influences on the ways in which practitioners identify and manage uncertainty and risks inherent in their efforts to develop their practice, which often places the individual practitioner and organization in a tenuous position. Strategies for moving practice forward within current health and social care policy, legal and professional frameworks for practice will be presented.

◯ Risk and risk perception in health care

The concept of risk has become prominent in our thoughts and touches all aspects of our lives (Hayes 1992). Many factors contribute to the prominence of risk in our personal and professional lives, such as the global impact of environmental disasters past, present and future (Beck 1992), advanced communication networks providing enhanced access and rapid transmission of events and knowledge, advancement of technology, bringing with it enormous benefits, as well as potential hazards, demographic and epidemiological trends, and growing antipathy toward the professionalization of risk analysis and risk management, particularly in situations where individuals manage complex, chronic diseases. This is the context in which practice is developed – an uncertain and constantly changing future.

An increased awareness of this context is needed to promote understanding of the ways in which risk knowledge contributes to the development of health care practice, and is translated into contemporary organizational strategies of risk management in the NHS in the United Kingdom. These issues are the focus of the latter section of this chapter. The initial discussion examines the nature of risk and risk construction, which will enable critical analysis of ways in which this knowledge is incorporated into these developments.

A range of definitions of risk can be found in the literature at the commencement of the twenty-first century. These definitions highlight attributes associated with risk, which tend to emphasize the negative aspects of risk, while discounting potential benefits resulting from risk-taking activities. These attributes include chance, possibility, probability, uncertainty, vulnerability, value, danger, hazard and peril. This negativity is illustrated in the Royal Society (1992: 2) definition of risk in health care, which states 'the probability that a particular adverse event occurs during a stated period of time, or results from a particular challenge'. This view suggests that risks can be objectively assessed. For example, potential violence in a health care setting can be assessed through identification and quantification of characteristics of the service user (for example history of violence, in pain, intoxication), the nurse (for example inexperienced, younger, poor communication skills) and circumstances relating to the service setting (such as waiting time, insufficient information, intrusion into personal privacy) (Poyner and Warne 1986). Although this information defines characteristics about the circumstances when violence is likely to occur, it cannot provide predictors with accuracy.

Heyman (1998) challenges the Royal Society view of risk on the grounds that it simplifies the complexity of events and reduces the influence of contributing factors. Furthermore, the focus is on the outcome of the event rather than locating the significance of the outcome in the values of individuals or social groups. For example, community nurses frequently work in isolated and potentially dangerous situations whilst providing care in home and community settings. In needle exchange services, nurses may work outside normal office hours, and act as the point of contact for drug users, sometimes in environments associated with high crime rates. Evaluation of the risks in these situations can be achieved through focusing on incidents of harm to practitioners, or the success of the service in accessing this client group. The focus of the evaluation contributes to shaping the outcome measures and in this case the results will differ. Alternatively, a pluralistic approach would seek to explore both perspectives in an endeavour to understand the range and significance of risks within the situation.

Risk communicators are poignantly aware that the attempt to present risk information as objective facts results in the presentation of only one piece of the puzzle. Morgan and Lave (1990: 357) highlight the importance of presenting multiple risk frames, stating that 'telling a risk story in only one way may mean telling it in a biased way. The only way to create a balanced impression may to be present several stories that present different framings or message formulation'. This in itself creates a dilemma because the story selection process is not a neutral act; it is implicitly value orientated. Johnson (1999) outlines the range of choices in this process, including the use of professional criteria (such as statistical data), audience preference (that is emotionally assuring concrete information) short-term versus long-term consequences, and local versus global consequences, to name a few. Thus risk construction is a product of the way in which risk knowledge is communicated, interpreted and acted on.

In health, complex and technical information is the cornerstone of professional knowledge; however, this is only one story. An alternative view of health is the way individuals manage their lives, in some situations accommodating complex changing states of disability and disease. For example, Clarke and Heyman (1998) present an account of the personal knowledge acquired by individuals who care for partners who are living with dementia, where the emphasis is not on technical knowledge of pathology, but on specific knowledge of the person. Such information may be denied to the professional. They identified that biographical knowledge, such as loss of self-identity of their partner and interpersonal concerns (such as loss of a life partner) were significant to carers. Clarke (2000) illustrates how these differing knowledge bases impact on risk perception, risk assessment and management in dementia care. This may result in contrasting views about the significance of potential events, such as falls or changing interpersonal relationships, influencing the way in which need is defined and care is shaped.

The relative value of these differing forms of knowledge is a major concern in contemporary health care. There remains, however, a dominance of professional over personal/lay knowledge. Furthermore, within the domain of professional knowledge there exists a hierarchy of evidence. For example, there is a trend in NHS policy to accept one kind of evidence, the randomized controlled trial (RCT), as closer to the truth about effective care. Kendall (1997) challenges the emphasis on this form of evidence, which provides the basis for prediction of events with limited explanatory power. She develops her argument on the basis of an analysis of the Oxford and Collaborators Health Check (OXCHECK 1995) study, which indicated that practice nurses were not as effective as predicted in making significant changes in coronary heart disease risk factors. Critical analysis of the limitations of the methodology of this study (RCT), and exploration of alternative methodologies led her to conclude that nurses working in primary care need to consider the meaning of evidence, and draw on evidence arising from different philosophical research positions to inform practice development. There is, however, a recognition of the need for more context-relevant research to be undertaken in the primary health care setting (NHS Executive 1997) which supports Kendall's argument, while recognizing immediate concerns about available, accessible evidence for practice. These professional debates are not new, but are being increasingly influenced by policy at a time when the nature of professional knowledge itself is argued to be more than understanding the scientific evidence. It includes the daily application of that knowledge, through reflecting on the outcomes of different actions (Benner 1984; Schön 1988; Closs and Cheater 1999).

The foregoing discussion attempted to provide an overview of risk construction and the complexity of risk knowledge, which discounts neither lay nor professional knowledge, while recognizing that tensions do exist. In situations where decisions about risk are made, consideration of risk knowledge is crucial but subject to a process of selective attention. This impacts on risk perception and the subsequent reaction to events. Heyman (1998) proposed that risk perception is influenced by the following factors.

1 *Risks must be identified.* For example, the relationship between lifting objects and potential back injury is now recognized. Prior to the identification of the causes of back injury, action to prevent injury could not be taken.

2 *Risks must be seen as controllable.* The way that risk messages are conveyed influences an individual's perception of the situation. Often information is given in the form of statistics of danger rather than a presentation of the safety margins, which impacts on the way that individuals make choices and see events as within their control (Heyman and Henriksen 2000). Furthermore, risks may be identified, yet the absence of perceived choice results in no action to modify or eliminate the potential harm. For example, until recently nurses regularly lifted clients in ways that could result in back injury, although the outcomes of poor handling practices were known. The nurses may have understood the potential hazards, yet lack of moving aids and features of the environment of care limited their ability to change their practice. It could be argued that increased compensation claims from injured nurses triggered health service managers to seek ways of preventing or minimizing such injuries to staff. Thus safe client handling techniques were developed. Hospital-style beds and specialized lifting equipment were made available in the home setting, enabling nurses to take action to minimize their personal risk of back injury, which had previously been accepted as an inevitable outcome of their work.

3 *Risks must be judged to have significant consequences.* Although actions may generate a range of consequences in any situation, individuals selectively emphasize those outcomes that they perceive to be important, and outcomes where they can exert some control over their circumstances to influence the attainment of their desired outcome (Heyman 1998).

Furthermore, the timescale of the impact of decisions is important – there may be long or short-term effects. Hence an individual may choose to emphasize the immediate implications of their decisions rather than future health outcomes. For example student nurses may understand the risks inherent in poor handling practices, yet they do lift in order to fit into the nursing team during their practice placement (Burgess 1996).

Differences in the selection of health and/or social consequences need to be appreciated when attempting to understand the rationale behind another's decision. Even when the rationale is understood, it may be judged to be of minimal significance and discounted. Table 4.1 identifies how risk is perceived.

Table 4.1   Risk perception

Risk perceptions are:
- to do with judgements, values, attitudes, and to do with decision making (not necessarily a rational process);
- are socially constructed;
- are politically negotiated.

Factors affecting risk perception include:
- perceived control over the situation;
- perceived losses and gains;
- perceived ability for protective actions;
- perceived susceptibility;
- perceived costs or barriers;
- availability influence;
- time and space;
- culture.

Such different perceptions of risk can be illustrated in diabetes care, where blood glucose control is emphasized by the professionals, while clients balance physiological concerns with other interests. For example, a taxi driver may experience great difficulty in complying with rigid dietary patterns, and opportunities for regular exercise may be minimal. This client, therefore, has a range of needs, including maintenance of physiological stability and continuing to carry out normal work. If the professional/client interaction focuses on assessing the effectiveness of treatment through monitoring of blood glucose and does not explore the experience of living with diabetes, this implicitly discounts the concerns and evaluations of the client (Watson and Heyman 1998).

Providing client defined care in an increasingly litigious society: a case study

The following case study exemplifies the way risk perception both defines and shapes care. Mrs Singleton has lived with Parkinson's disease for approximately 12 years. During the last three years she has experienced increasing mobility problems, difficulties in meeting her personal needs and extreme limitations in contributing to maintenance of the home. Her husband has been able to meet her increasing physical needs with no support from health or social care agencies. They are fiercely resistant to losing their independence, although the husband's burden of caring is beginning to contribute to emotional and physical problems.

The escalating needs in this situation came to a crisis point when the husband had to be admitted to a local hospital as an emergency patient with a condition that necessitated surgery. Relatives and neighbours were able to provide care for Mrs Singleton through arrangement of a rota. Following symptom relief and assessment, it was agreed that Mr Singleton could return home prior to planned surgery in four days' time. The care provided for Mrs Singleton had met her immediate needs, however, it was doubtful that this arrangement could be sustained during the convalescence period of approximately six weeks following Mr Singleton's surgery. These concerns were discussed with the medical and nursing team, and arrangements were made for the medical social worker to visit Mr and Mrs Singleton to explore available options to meet their needs.

Various options were discussed, including provision of aids to enhance Mrs Singleton's ability to move independently and organization of a short-term placement in a nursing home for Mrs Singleton. The couple were aware of each other's immediate physical needs, but they were also concerned about the escalation of care provision which they had resisted for a considerable time. The risks in this situation were very real to all of the participants in this scenario. For example, providing aids and additional support, such as the provision of a care assistant to help Mrs Singleton to bathe, may have enabled her to meet the most pressing physical needs. This level of support would have enabled the couple to remain together and retain a level of independence which they valued. This arrangement may, however, have increased the potential of other risks, such as Mrs Singleton falling and sustaining physical harm (she had a history of falls and injury), and Mr Singleton exposing himself to post-operative complications as a consequence of moving his wife throughout the day and night.

An alternative analysis of this situation may focus on the responsibilities of the relevant professionals. Should they prioritize the maximization of safety, that is physical safety in this situation (which may result in moving the location of care to a nursing home) at the expense of the emotional and social needs of this couple and their desired course of action? Norman (1980) suggested that the main concern of professional care involves protecting clients from harm which, in many circumstances, is interpreted as prioritizing potential physical harm in relation to other harms.

If the professionals focused the plan of care around this couple's interpersonal needs and desire to remain in their home, they would require support that could be provided through innovative service reconfiguration and flexible role negotiation, such as the use of community support workers. However, if either partner sustained physical injury, attention would be drawn to this situation by the couple, the employing organization and the wider community, and the professionals may have found themselves in the rather uncomfortable position of defending their actions and facing potential negligence charges. Although these outcomes may seem extreme in this fictional case, it does serve the purpose of

illustrating some of the factors that influence perception of risk in practice and subsequent appraisal of the outcomes of events.

The importance of the client's perspective in risk assessment and management has been stressed throughout the previous discussion and is
implicit in the subsequent exploration of practice development where
the focus will centre on practitioner concerns.

◯ Patients, services, need and risk

Nursing care has changed substantially during the 1990s in response to
health policy, changing organizational structures and alteration in professional guidance to identify a few key drivers. The UKCC document
The Scope of Professional Practice (UKCC 1992a) was one influential initiative that provided a vehicle for expansion and development of nursing
roles. Alongside the opportunity for role enhancement, an awareness of
unmet client need identified through sustained contact with the client
group, awareness of shortcomings in current practice and enhanced understanding of alternative ways of providing services, created the impetus
for nurses and other professionals to change their practice (Clarke *et al.*
1998). Thus the emergence of new roles enabled nurses to respond to
client need in new and innovative ways.

Implicit in the development of new roles is the challenge of managing
complementary, yet potentially competing demands of promoting client
safety and developing practice. Client safety is promoted through well-
planned strategies, which are implemented to minimize potential harm
and maximize effective outcomes. Although consistent with these aims,
the outcomes of new practices are by their very nature uncertain. The
potential to enhance quality of care exists, however the challenge is to
limit the possibility that outcomes will deteriorate. Thus, practice development creates circumstances where the practitioner, client and organization are exposed to potential risks. Risk issues inherent in practice
development can be summarized as:

- actual/potential harms and benefits (to clients, practitioner and
  organization);
- identification and development of skills and competencies to meet the
  demands of new roles and new ways of working (education and training requirements);
- delegation of normal duties;
- communication and documentation considerations;
- enhancing and going beyond the scope of existing practice;
- negotiation of roles (for instance, nurses feeling pressured to take on
  roles beyond their individual competencies);
- negotiation of the parameters for autonomous decision making;

- defining standards of care;
- defining responsibility and accountability in enhanced roles and new practices;
- clarifying legal parameters for the development and change of practice;
- client perceptions about customary roles, such as the role of a GP, and the new role-holder, such as a practice nurse;
- organizational commitment to new roles/services;
- interdisciplinary and/or interagency collaboration;
- environment of care;
- maintenance of equipment and development of competence to use the equipment (particularly new equipment in the practice setting);
- managing the process of change;
- outcome measurement and evaluation.

This is an impressive and daunting list to consider prior to developing any aspect of practice. It would, however, be unwise for any professional to embark on changing practice without giving due consideration to each of these issues. It is beyond the scope of this chapter to explore each of these issues in depth; therefore, examination of three themes implicit within each of these issues, are discussed to promote consideration of uncertainties and risks inherent in developing practice.

◯ Standards of practice

All professionals owe their clients a duty of care, which implies that practice standards are shaped by professions drawing on and responding to current knowledge, policy and law, to name but a few influences. The principles underpinning practice standards in nursing are embodied in the UKCC *Code of Professional Conduct for Nurses, Midwives and Health Visitors* (1992b). This document seeks to explicate the highest professional standards that the professional translates to their own practice. Alternatively, legal standards indicate the minimum level below which practice must not fall. It is therefore useful to explore the minimum requirements, which determines the baseline for further development.

In English law, the standard of care required of a health professional was established in a case in 1957 called Bolam v Frien Hospital Management Committee.[1] Here, it was stated by the judge that a doctor (could be replaced by nurse)[2] is not guilty of negligence 'if he has acted in accordance with a practice accepted as proper by a responsible body of medical men skilled in that particular area' (Bolam v Frien Hospital Management Committee 1957: 582).

This has come to be known as the Bolam test. Essentially, this test indicates that professionals are to be judged against the practice standards of their peers. Although this case refers to the skills 'of an ordinary competent man' (which can be replaced by 'nurse') it is reasonable to assume that individuals who have particular specialized skills will be able to perform particular tasks with greater expertise. For example, enhanced knowledge about asthma and its management, respiratory assessment skills and patient education would be amongst the skills and abilities required of a nurse working as a specialist practitioner in an asthma clinic.

It is important to note that individuals who are developing and expanding their roles will be expected to meet the standards normally required of the post holder, albeit a general practitioner. Increasingly, nurse practitioners in general practice assess and diagnose health problems, or hold pre-assessment clinics for planned surgery. In these situations, the competence of the nurse will be compared to doctors who are the normal role holder. In Wilsher v Essex Area Health Authority (1986) arguments by the defendants, that the junior doctors did their best in view of their inexperience, was rejected. It was upheld that the obligation on professionals was to meet the standards of competence and experience from those fulfilling demanding roles.

Thus the minimal legal requirement is for practitioners to implement approved or accepted standards in their practice. Generally, accepted practice is that which is widely spread within the profession at a particular point in time. Practices, however, do differ and differences will continue to exist, but this is acceptable. For example, in Maynard v West Midlands Regional Health Authority (1984: 634) Lord Scarman stated that 'a judge's preference for one distinguished professional opinion to another also professionally distinguished is not sufficient to establish negligence in a practitioner'.

Thus any recognized practice may be followed. More recently, there have been situations where the Bolam test has been contested as the test to be applied when determining practice standards. For example, in the Bolitho (1998) case a senior paediatric registrar failed to attend a child with respiratory difficulties. The child suffered a cardiac arrest and sustained serious brain damage. A key issue in this case was causation and the Bolam principle. The case went to the Court of Appeal and House of Lords where Lord Browne-Wilkinson stated:

> the use of these adjectives responsible, reasonable and respectable all show that the court has to be satisfied that the exponents of the body of opinion relied upon can demonstrate that such opinion has a logical basis. In particular, in cases involving, as they often do, the weighing of risks against benefits, the judge before accepting a body of opinion as being responsible, reasonable or respectable, will need to be satisfied that, in forming their views, the experts have directed

their minds to the question of comparative risks and benefits and have reached a defensible conclusion on the matter.

(Bolitho v City and Hackney Health Authority 1998: 33)

Tingle (1998) argued that this case will have implications for expert reports, guideline/procedure/protocol development and evidence-based medicine and nursing. It also addresses the complexity of standards in practice, and the nature of the evidence which determines contemporary practice standards.

Practice development by its very purpose seeks to change what currently exists and to depart from current accepted standards. If patients are harmed through the outcomes of new practices, there may be few defences to support the practitioner. Thus practitioners may be guarded about changing what is acceptable and placing themselves in a vulnerable position. This would result in stagnation and limited quality enhancement of practice. Departure from accepted practice is recognized in law, in circumstances where it can be demonstrated that there are strong reasons to change practice. For example, research findings indicate that cleansing of open traumatic wounds (Riyat and Quinton 1997) and of acute traumatic soft tissue wounds (Angeras *et al.* 1992) with tap water, creates no higher rate of infection than cleansing with sterile saline, and has considerable cost savings.

Practitioners must also be mindful that there may be risks inherent in refraining from developing their practice. Clarke *et al.* (1998) identified that the impetus for practice development in many situations is located in the identification of unmet client need. Therefore clients may be exposed to known harms through failure to respond to their need by continuing to provide customary services.

In circumstances where practices are changed, a duty would be placed on the practitioner to take precautions against foreseeable untoward events. Lord Denning, in Roe v Minister of Health (1954), acknowledged that medical and nursing practices resulted in benefits and risks to the client. This results in an obligation to minimize harms and maximize benefits to the client, which is complementary to the aims of practice development. In many circumstances, potential and actual harms are not foreseeable at the outset of changing practice and role development. Caution therefore should be exercised when planning a move from accepted practice, through the use of systematic, regular monitoring mechanisms to constantly evaluate client/service outcomes and adverse events.

◯ Risk identification and assessment

Risks in health care have been broadly categorized as those relating to direct patient care (such as risks relating to standards of care), indirect patient care (such as security risks, fire risks, risk arising from waste), health and safety (for example unsafe systems of work, control of substances hazardous to health) and organizational considerations (like communication and information systems failure) (NHS Management Executive 1993). The two main approaches used in health care, to identify the range of risks related to staff, clients and resources, are risk assessment strategies and clinical incident reporting.

These approaches are complementary, providing information about situations that have occurred, or may occur in the future, to support actions designed to minimize or eliminate the identified risk. Thus the robustness of information used to inform risk management processes, is crucial to the development of comprehensive and viable plans. Acquisition of relevant information is, however, problematic. For example, reporting of clinical incidents may underrepresent the frequency of actual incidents, when staff are concerned that they may face disciplinary action on the basis of the information provided. These factors should be carefully considered when making decisions about future practices and management structures.

Clinical risk assessment is a proactive process whereby information is collected and analysed to identify aspects of care which fall below acceptable standards, and acquiring knowledge of the reasons for this occurrence. This is achieved through exploration of data acquired from a range of sources, such as clinical audit, client and staff satisfaction surveys, individual staff interviews, staff group discussion, client complaints, clinical incident reports, claims data, risk assessment tools, clinical indicators and comparative data acquired from elsewhere (Walshe and Dineen 1998). Analysis of this information will provide knowledge about the intensity, frequency and significance of actual and potential untoward events.

The type and frequency of risks vary considerably across health care practice, reflecting characteristics of the practice, practice setting and needs of the client group. For example, in community nursing there are specific hazards relating to the location of the practice, such as in the client's home, or other environments within the community, which are outside the direct control of the trust. Data sources used to identify risks vary, and in many instances, context-specific risk assessment tools have been developed to identify the general and specific risks in the practice and location of care (see Table 4.2). In this tool, specific hazards are identified in the first column, a detailed analysis of high-risk situations and potential outcomes are identified in the second column, and planned actions to modify the risk are presented in the third. This tool is used to identify and manage hazards faced by community nurses in this practice setting.

In some situations, knowledge about untoward events may have been the impetus for considering developments in practice. This is illustrated

Table 4.2   Risk assessment tool
Two examples from a generic assessment.

Hazard	Risks	Controls
Violence to staff	• personal injury to staff who are at risk of violence while at work; • risk is greatest for lone workers, those handling cash or drugs, and staff dealing with irate members of the public or difficult patients; • civil litigation could result if the trust negligently places staff at risk of violence.	• Community staff are to leave planned timetable of visits at their base and report in periodically. • High risk patient/areas are to be identified and staff notified. • When required, staff are to be provided with personal attack alarms or mobile phones. • No unaccompanied visits are to be allowed to high risk patients, who are to be seen at health centres/clinics whenever possible. • Panic buttons are to be fitted in high risk areas. • No member of staff is to be left alone on the premises at times when the public has access. • The layout of furniture in interview/treatment rooms is to ensure staff have access to means of escape in the event of a violent incident.
Home visits	• risk of injury to staff faced with violent incidents in the patient's home; • risk of injury to staff and patients due to lack of lifting aids in the home environment; • risk of injury to staff due to tripping hazards in the patients home; • risk of injury associated with the transportation of gas cylinders and clinical waste in cars.	• Staff undertaking home visits must make their own assessment of the risks present in each patient's home. • Where risks are present, staff should follow the guidance contained in the relevant section of this generic risk assessment. • Where risks are deemed to be high, staff should contact their manager for advice on how to proceed.

in Amanda's story (Box 4.1), where knowledge of difficulties and potentially dangerous delays encountered by patients attempting to access emergency medical care during the night, led to the development of nurses' clinical assessment skills to assess and triage patients to the appropriate level of emergency care. Therefore, analysis of data sources which provide information about the outcomes of current practice and service provision may indicate areas where improvements could be made, or highlight alternative ways to meet client need, as well as contributing to the process of risk identification and assessment.

In addition to providing a rationale for developing existing practice, this information also provides a rationale for departing from current accepted practice, which would be required in situations where clients were harmed and sought redress. Further analysis of this practice data facilitates identification of foreseeable risks, and this may be used to stimulate the development of strategies to minimize the potential harms. One of the foreseeable risks in innovative practices is the potential for unknown outcomes; therefore, it would be incumbent on practitioners to develop evaluation strategies alongside new initiatives to provide continuous feedback about the impact of the new service, and propose changes where new risks to clients, staff and the organization are identified.

Commentary

Amanda's story illustrates some of the risks and difficulties encountered in role expansion and the development of new services. It highlights the importance of developing approaches to elicit knowledge of user satisfaction with existing services, unmet patient need and developing an understanding of existing and planned changes to practitioner roles. Thus development of a comprehensive understanding of the situation and identification of risks implicit in changes to existing services is essential prior to implementing the changes in practice.

Professional guidance from the UKCC (1992a) provides a framework for nurses such as Amanda to develop and expand their roles. The document *The Scope of Professional Practice* (UKCC 1992a) emphasizes the need to maintain and develop patient-focused practice through role expansion, while not compromising existing service provision or resulting in inappropriate delegation (Scholefield *et al.* 1997). This guidance stresses professional accountability, and the need to maintain and develop knowledge, skills and competence that are appropriate to the new role.

To minimize identified risks in this situation, customized training and education programmes were drawn up to develop competencies that were required in the new role. For example, the programmes aimed to expand the nurses' existing skills in carrying out holistic assessment through developing complementary skills of taking a medically focused assessment.

Box 4.1   Amanda's story: responding to client need through the development of an 'out of hours' district nursing service

As an experienced district nurse working on the night nursing service, I was aware of the difficulties encountered by patients in accessing appropriate health care advice and emergency medical care outside normal surgery hours. I observed frequent long delays in the attendance of a doctor from the deputizing service who provided emergency medical care. In many cases, it would be neither appropriate nor practical for patients to attend an accident and emergency department, or an emergency primary care centre. I reflected on these difficulties and considered the feasibility of the night nursing service offering an accessible contact point for patients to get advice, assessment or referral.

A survey was carried out to identify the frequency and severity of the problem. I also attended conferences about out of hours primary care developments in the UK, which further stimulated my interest and belief that there were practical ways to develop existing services to provide more patient focused care during the night. I put forward a proposal to the community services manager for a project to expand the function of the out of hours nursing service. These plans included provision of telephone triage and advanced clinical assessment by nurses for patients requiring access to medical services outside normal surgery hours. Following initial assessment, patients would be treated by the staff in the new nursing service or referred to the GP or hospital.

It was anticipated that the service would provide enhanced patient-focused care and reduce delays in accessing health advice. In addition, inappropriate referrals to the accident and emergency department may be reduced, and the work of the overnight medical staff in primary care may then focus on the more urgent health problems.

As part of a university course, I underwent training in advanced clinical assessment and developed the skills of taking medically focused patient histories, and carrying out physical assessment, such as chest auscultation and abdominal palpation. The training needs of the other nurses operating the service also included enhanced clinical assessment training. With the support of management and a local GP practice, a pilot study for the out of hours nursing service was carried out.

Three months following commencement of the pilot study, an evaluation was conducted. The findings indicated that there was a high level of patient satisfaction with the new service, and the nursing staff suggested that the service was an appropriate first point of contact for patients during the night. Furthermore, the nurses indicated that they had experienced an increase in their job satisfaction, which was attributed to further development of their knowledge and skills in clinical assessment. The enhanced skills contributed to the attainment of high standards of patient assessment and referral to other services where necessary. The GPs were also satisfied that the needs of their patients were being met. Consequently, the trust agreed to support an extended trial of the out of hours nursing service.

Thus the nurses developed skills to enable them to communicate the need for urgent referral to the appropriate service. The programme also focused on enhancing their existing decision making skills and planning abilities. These existing and new skills addressed the myriad of influences that affect patients in their home environments, which is a characteristic of community nursing practice identified by other authors (for example Bryans and McIntosh 1996).

Changes to the nurses' roles affected other professionals working in this primary care setting, as well as the users of the service. They were incorporating some aspects of the customary role of the medical staff, which required careful negotiation with the doctors. Also, the patients' expectations of the usual role holder may have been at variance to the proposals in the new service; therefore, their views needed consideration. One way to address these issues was the implementation of a communication system within the team and with users of the service to promote an understanding of the role and service development. Furthermore, ongoing monitoring of the outcomes of the service was designed to provide information about the effectiveness of changes to provision, and enable the identification of risks that had not been considered prior to the commencement of the project.

◯ Risk-taking and risk modification

The aim of risk identification is to promote change in practice, or to institute plans alongside new developments, to enhance the quality of care and minimize potential harm. In some situations, the objectives of care and treatment are inseparable from the inherent risks. This is highlighted in the case of Mr and Mrs Singleton, where maintaining support for the couple in the community does not limit the potential for falls and injury, while the therapeutic value of maintaining their independence is obvious.

Such risk-taking activities are inherent in many aspects of practice, such as rehabilitation following stroke, self-medication and self-care programmes to enhance the possibility of obtaining beneficial outcomes. In these situations, it would be unreasonable to neglect plans to minimize potential harms, such as over or underdoses in the case of self-medication. Reasonable plans may include spot checks on compliance with the medication regime (Ryan 1993). Likewise, avoiding strategically planned risk-taking in practice inhibits the maximization of beneficial outcomes to the client. These situations present dilemmas for practitioners, particularly against a background of increasing litigation. In these situations, actions that would reduce the risks to the practitioner in the event of harm to clients include:

- in-depth analysis of harms and benefits in the plan of care;
- negotiation of the plan of care with the client exploring risks and benefits;
- development of safeguards to reduce harmful outcomes;
- accurate and detailed recording of decisions, including justification of the decision in the light of current practice and knowledge;
- accurate and detailed recording in the care plan to provide evidence that care had been taken in the planning of care.

(Cook 1996)

Alternatively, there are many situations where circumstances, environment or behaviour can be changed, resulting in minimization or elimination of health care risk. This is known as risk modification (Wilson 1995; Wilson and Tingle 1999). Analysis of the identified risk(s) will highlight features of the situation where problems occur and ways to customize risk modification plans to the practice setting. For example,

- guidance may be required for using new equipment;
- training put in place to develop knowledge and skills to undertake new roles/practices;
- policy implemented for acquiring informed consent to treatment;
- issuing staff with mobile phones/alarms, when working in dangerous or unsafe environments;
- protocols developed for providing blood transfusion services at home.

The effectiveness of these plans should be subjected to evaluation, leading to improvement in the quality of service provision. Alongside in-depth analysis of the situation and planning to minimize potential harm, it is essential that the rationale for the planned actions, care and/ or service development is carefully documented to provide a systematic, comprehensive and accurate record of the event. This record will be essential if problems do occur; indeed, it may serve as a defence for the actions that were taken. These issues are further explored in Harry's story (Box 4.2).

Commentary

The commentary on the scenario in Box 4.2 will focus on the use of guidelines to modify the risks in this situation. Approaches to practice vary, and there was concern in this situation that there should be agreement between all of the professionals who would be involved with the new service to clarify practice standards and minimize potential variation in practice. Von Degenberg (1996) suggests that the process of

Box 4.2   Harry's story: organizational risks in the use of home blood transfusion

As a district nurse of many years' experience, I have often felt that the need for patients to be hospitalized overnight in order to be given a routine blood transfusion was an unnecessary upheaval in their lives, when they were already coping with the stresses of living with chronic illness. After carrying out an extensive literature review, I learned that there were areas of the UK where blood transfusions were carried out at home, with the support of the primary care team and trained auxiliary nurses. I discussed the feasibility of a home transfusion service with the general practitioners, who were very supportive and interested in developing the idea further.

Although the idea potentially had great benefits to individual patients, I was aware that the proposed service would be viewed as a 'high risk' activity by the trust in which I worked. In order to enhance my understanding of the need for this type of service, and the difficulties which may be encountered in developing and implementing the service, I discussed the idea with my community nurse manager, the trust risk assessment coordinator and the haematology consultant. They agreed that the proposed service would be beneficial to patients, and I gained support for a small pilot project. I completed an extensive risk assessment, and identified several concerns, including transport of the blood to the home, disposal of equipment following the transfusion, competence of staff to implement and monitor the procedure, and access to emergency services in the event of a reaction to the blood during the transfusion.

Plans were developed to address every issue identified in the risk assessment. For example,

- transportation of blood – a cool box was purchased to carry the blood from the hospital to the patient's home. In the pilot study, it was agreed that I would check the blood at the hospital using the standard checking procedure and take it to the patient's home;
- disposal of equipment – the trust's policy on disposal of contaminated products from the patient's home would be followed;
- competence of staff – a training needs analysis was undertaken for the auxiliary nurse and myself. Training packages were arranged to develop our competence to fulfil our roles which included:
  - qualified nurse: implementation, monitoring and terminating the blood transfusion;
  - auxiliary nurse: monitoring the blood transfusion;
- delegation of duties – guidelines were developed to indicate duties that could be delegated and the scope of the role of the auxiliary nurse;
- standards of practice – multiprofessional guidelines were negotiated to indicate the standards of practice that were required and to provide clarification of staff roles and responsibilities;
- emergency contact – a mobile phone was purchased to ensure that direct contact between service staff and emergency services could be maintained;

- medical support – negotiation with one of the general practitioners resulted in providing medical support for the new service.

Following preparation, the first patient was identified for the pilot study. He was a gentleman of 63 years who suffered from leukaemia. He had a severe dislike of the hospital setting and was keen to take part in the project.

I carried out the cannulation and started the transfusion with no difficulty in the patient's home at 10 a.m. The procedure was progressing normally and I left to continue with other nursing duties in the community. The nursing auxiliary remained in the home to monitor the blood transfusion. Prior to leaving the house, I checked that the mobile telephone was working and she had my contact number and the number for the relevant general practitioner for emergency backup. I arranged to return regularly to the house to check progress throughout the four hours of the procedure.

drawing up guidelines facilitates the identification of appropriate, effective and efficient care and the use of agreed guidelines reduces unacceptable variation in clinical practice. The process of developing guidelines can also promote multidisciplinary understanding and agreement about treatment, which is crucial in this situation where the procedure requires multiprofessional collaboration and coordination of activities across the primary secondary interface to ensure that the patient receives the blood transfusion.

The quality of guidelines is important. They should be evidence-based and be specific to the needs of the patient and the user. Conroy and Shannon (1995) suggest that guidelines, which are developed from an analysis of current evidence, can set out the optimum management approach for a given condition. Guidelines, however, are tools to inform clinical decision making, and the quality of the decision will be influenced by the competence of the practitioner. Overreliance on guidelines may lead to non-questioning practice (Flanagan 1997), which may not fully meet the needs of the patient. Therefore guidelines should include recommendations for the standards of practice for the blood transfusion, while providing a framework whereby clinical judgement can be exercised to assess the cannulation site or the significance of mild pyrexia.

Guidelines have been advocated as a risk management and quality assurance mechanism (Tingle 1995; Von Degenberg 1996) because they provide written evidence of the agreed standard of care, and demonstrate that the professionals thought proactively about the care given. The standards of care articulated in the guidelines provide a quality framework against which to measure practice (RCN 1995). In this situation, the measurement of the practice would contribute to evaluation and review of service processes and outcomes.

⭕ Organizational strategies for risk management

The emphasis in the previous discussion has focused on the practitioner's constraints and responsibilities for identifying and managing risk in their practice, with minimal reference to the wider organizational context. This context will have risk management frameworks that should both inform and be informed by any changes in service provision. Therefore the final discussion in this chapter will provide a brief overview of corporate risk management in contemporary health care.

The organizational approach to risk in health care services developed initially as a means of controlling litigation, which has been a major concern in the United States since the mid-1970s, and a growing problem in the UK for at least since the late 1980s (both in quantity of cases and rising awards for damages). This origin resulted in a restricted conceptualization of risk management which is both negative and defensive. This view suggests that the primary aim of risk management is to focus on protection of the trust from claims, with little regard to the origin of those claims, or for the well-being of the patients concerned. An extended conceptualization of risk management is positive, and includes the emphasis on improving the quality of care and reducing the incidence of harm (Vincent 1995). Thus the need to consider underlying clinical problems becomes apparent.

Until recently in the UK the responsibility for managing clinical risk was left to the clinicians, including self-regulation of the quality of practice. However there has been a perceptible shift from the emphasis on professional self-regulation, where a presumption of competence is paramount, towards a requirement that fitness to practice should be constantly reassessed through a process of reaccreditation (Walshe and Dineen 1998). This movement has been influenced by recent health care problems where multisystem failures and poor quality care have been reported. In many of these instances, there have been multiple mistakes in a chain of error, which could have been avoided if effective clinical risk management systems were in place (Wilson and Tingle 1997).

The risk management process is a systematic and comprehensive review of services and systems in an organization. It includes the following interrelated stages:

- risk assessment and risk identification – this is the process by which the organization becomes aware of potential or actual harm to service users and staff (see previous discussion);
- risk analysis – the measurement of risk and the impact it has on the organization (assessing the level and severity, expectancy and frequency of identified risks);

- risk reduction and control decisions – implementing changes to clinical and organizational practices, so that adverse events are eliminated or made less likely; in the event of actual harm the focus is on immediate action to address client need;
- risk funding recognizing that some adverse events will happen, and ensuring that costs of such events are both minimized and provided for, through good claims management and adequate insurance or other cover.

(Walshe and Dineen 1998)

In the NHS the development of clinical risk management is part of a wider move towards greater corporate accountability for performance, which initially focused on financial concerns. DoH (1997c) guidance attempted to clarify organizational responsibilities, which included financial issues, estates and non-clinical risk, whereas the White Paper *The New NHS: Modern, Dependable* (DoH 1997a) extended the process of corporate accountability to issues of clinical performance, and introduced the concept of clinical governance (DoH 1998d). This guidance located the statutory duty for quality maintenance and improvement in health care with NHS boards and those who lead them. Hence, the government required NHS trusts to embrace the concept of clinical governance which creates a framework through which NHS organizations are accountable for continuously improving the quality of their services (DoH 1997a, 1998d).

Many of the systems required in clinical governance already exist, including clinical risk management, claims management and the identification and handling of adverse events in clinical care. The new emphasis is on integrating these disparate systems. This agenda is supported by specific commitment to new structures and systems designed to measure and improve quality such as The National Institute for Clinical Excellence (NICE) and the Commission for Health Improvement (CHI)[3]. These developments are intended to provide frameworks to promote evidence-based practice, thereby promoting certainty and creating safety for the client and the organization.

Procter (1999) suggests that practice is defined in the approach promoted in contemporary health policy as technical competence, and challenges the dominance of this approach on the basis that it focuses on narrow, unidimensional definitions of health care outcomes. She proposes that acceptance of alternative models of practice development, such as action research and practitioner enquiry, may embrace broad definitions of clinical effectiveness and experiential and contextual practice knowledge, while engaging with diverse perspectives of risk construction. In this model, practice development may synthesize multiple perspectives in health care, resulting in contextual knowledge rather than decontextualized knowledge. This may be more appropriate to decision making processes about the particular clinical setting. These proposals promote an alternative way of developing practice at a time when clients are seeking a health service that is able to respond effectively at the point of need.

◯ Taking practice forward

Taking and managing risk is a central part of developing practice. Although it is anticipated that the results of the new practice will enhance the quality of existing practice and service provision, the very nature of practice development creates a situation where outcomes are uncertain. Positive outcomes such as the development of appropriate, effective and efficient client care are welcomed, however, there is limited tolerance of untoward outcomes. In the latter circumstances, there has been an increased emphasis on medical negligence. One set of responses to this situation in health care has been a focus on risk management in the NHS, that is, the identification, modification or elimination of risk. The danger of the current emphasis on risk in health care is the response from practitioners, who may avoid engaging in situations where uncertainty is predominant, such as practice development. The consequences for clients and the service may, however, be detrimental in the long term, through the loss of creativity and innovation in practice. There is the emergence of a paradox in contemporary health care for professionals: at a time when there are immense opportunities for role expansion and practice development, they work in a context where there is minimal tolerance of uncertain practice outcomes.

The argument developed in this chapter is that practitioners should strive to continually develop their practice. This cannot, however, occur haphazardly. Practitioners are responsible for careful planning of new initiatives to promote positive and minimize negative outcomes. This can be facilitated through comprehensive assessment of risk, which includes user, professional and organizational perspectives. The risks that are identified during this process should be analysed to inform plans to modify or eliminate the harms. This approach will not stifle innovation; instead, it provides a framework to promote safe practice development.

◯ Notes

1 See the list of cases at the end of this chapter.
2 The authors' inclusion; see Samuels (1993).
3 NICE is responsible for assessing the clinical and cost-effectiveness of new technologies and producing recommendations and guidelines for the NHS.

CHI is charged with the responsibility to ensure that NHS organizations have adequate clinical governance arrangements in place and to intervene where necessary to tackle quality problems.

◯ List of cases

Bolitho v City and Hackney Health Authority (1998) *Lloyd's Reports Medical*, 26.

Bolam v Frien Hospital Management Committee (1957) 1 WLR 582; (1957) 1 *Butterworths Medical Legal Reports*, 1.

Maynard v West Midlands Regional Health Authority (1985) 1 *All England Law Reports* 635; (1984) 1 WLR 634.

Roe v Minister of Health [1954] 2 *Queens Bench* 66.

Wilsher v Essex Area Health Authority (1986) 3 *All England Law Reports* 801, Court of Appeal.

⑤ Education for change

Sue Spencer

◯ Chapter summary

This chapter seeks to debate whether higher education acts as an ally or an adversary during the development of practice. The notion that educational institutions have a legitimate and unproblematic relationship with the development of nursing practice is critically reviewed. In the chapter, the role that higher education can and does play within practice development is articulated together with an appraisal of the potential hazards and pitfalls which such an approach may present.

◯ Community nursing and higher education in the twenty-first century

In 1994, the UKCC determined that the specialist area of community nursing should be developed at first degree level (UKCC 1994). This new unified discipline of community health care specialist practitioner identifies transferable core competencies amongst:

- general practice nursing;
- community mental health nursing;
- community learning disabilities nursing;
- community children's nursing;
- public health nursing/health visiting;
- occupational health nursing;
- nursing in the home/district nursing;
- school nursing.

These competencies are:

- the ability to monitor and improve standards of care;
- supervision of practice;
- clinical audit;
- developing and leading practice;
- research-based practice and research activity.

This integrated approach has proved to be a challenge for students, lecturers and existing practitioners alike. There now exists a dichotomy between the 'new' specialist community practitioner and those 'old' practitioners, with traditional or no community qualifications. In the early years, transitional arrangements were made for community nurses to gain recognition as specialist practitioners, but these have been accessed predominantly by district and practice nursing. The newer community specialist, with no history of mandatory postregistration qualifications such as learning disabilities and school nursing, has been left behind in relation to continuing professional development.

This very brief overview of the relationship between community nursing provides two areas for further debate for practitioners and clinical managers. The first issue concerns the personal and professional development of existing non-graduate practitioners. Confronted with the new breed of graduate community nurse, they may feel (and have felt) undermined and undervalued. Educational opportunities may be scarce, as the necessity for resources to be concentrated in creating newly qualified practitioners means that little time and money are left for those already qualified. Given that many of these practitioners are required to supervise and mentor newly qualified graduates, it is ironic that employers and universities do not feel that they should invest in these people's development.

The second issue is the provision of appropriate continuing professional development for the graduate specialist practitioner. Some have seen the next step as embracing expanded roles that encroach into medical roles. This has created a great deal of debate and analysis about the implications of this expanded role and the impact on roles and relationships within the community. It has also proved to be a challenge to higher education to provide educational opportunities that develop practitioners and utilize the skills and knowledge they have developed in their first degrees.

There would appear to be much more potential for making a link between continuing professional development with the development of practice. This issue is addressed later in this chapter. By responding to cues from practice, practitioners may be more able to identify for themselves the educational experiences they wish to access. They should be able to clearly identify the structure and content of the course that will enhance their practice, rather than access education solely for the piece of paper.

Before we examine the problematic nature of higher education's involvement in practice development, it is important that we examine the ways in which students, and indeed their teachers, may be involved in such developments. Unsworth (2000) identifies that professional development plays a major part in most developments in practice. He asserts that professional development can occur as an antecedent to practice development. For example, attendance at a course of study may trigger the practitioner to seek to introduce changes in the way they deliver that aspect of care (Allison 1995). Professional development may also be part of the process of practice development. For example, it may be necessary to teach practitioners to perform a new skill to improve an aspect of practice, like compression bandaging. Finally, professional development can be a consequence of practice development. For example, if a practitioner wanted to change an aspect of practice and undertook a literature search as part of the process, then the practitioner would have developed professionally as a result.

Clearly, higher education faces a challenge to provide education and professional development activities that are able to support practitioners to develop practice. Essentially, higher education plays several different but complementary roles in supporting the development of practice. These include:

- standard setter and promoter of 'best practice';
- information disseminator;
- enabler;
- professional developer.

◯ Promotion of 'best practice' and information disseminator

The student as a change agent

Higher education, together with NHS service providers, is jointly responsible for identifying and assessing the competence of both preregistration and postregistration practitioners. This, together with a desire on the part of teachers to promote best practice, goes some way towards setting the standards of practice, albeit indirectly. While such an approach is admirable, it is not without its problems. Nurse teachers are not usually in a position to directly influence the delivery of care. As a result, the temptation is either to enable practitioners to identify what needs to change, and equip them with the skills and knowledge to make that change happen, or to seek to use the student as an agent of change.

This scenario occurs frequently in the case of preregistration students, and can be seen when the student encounters difficulties about poor or inappropriate practice while on placement. Students often raise these issues when they return to the university, and the response they receive is that they should raise their concerns with the staff concerned. This has in the past led to students being labelled as difficult and resulted in some animosity between ward staff and students. Similar problems can occur for postregistration students, although the response and the student's ability to deal with it and produce meaningful developments in practice, differs according to a number of factors. Principal amongst these factors are seniority and the length of time the student has worked in the clinical area. More senior staff, or those who have worked in a clinical setting for several years, are likelier to be able to innovate than those who are in junior positions.

Students who are studying for a specialist practitioner qualification are in a more difficult position. While many of these practitioners are experienced, they are often new to the area of specialist practice, and this makes them dependent upon others for guidance about what aspect of practice to develop and how to go about it. As a result, students are often forced to develop an area of practice effectively selected for them because it is manageable and of interest to the students' practice teacher. Other issues of concern include:

- saving developments for the student to do during their course;
- giving the student the practice teacher's pet project;
- novice students attempting to fit their past clinical experience into a new environment, for example concentrating on cardiac disease because of past experience in coronary care;
- overambitious projects that require organizational change, rather than solely dependent on a discrete group of practitioners in a particular setting.

Lynn's story (Box 5.1) illustrates some of the tensions that can occur when using educational courses to develop practice. Lynn was new to health visiting when she joined the course, having previously worked in the intensive therapy unit (ITU). Effectively Lynn was an expert nurse who had been reduced to a novice because of the change to her area of practice. This move is difficult enough without having to cope with the increased stresses of deciding upon an area of clinical practice to develop within six weeks of starting the course. In effect, the nature of her higher education programme was forcing her to decide what aspect of health visiting practice to develop before she had even begun to learn what health visiting was really about. The outcome of the first meeting between the lecturer and the practice teacher was that the practice teacher had already decided upon the area of practice that Lynn should

---

Box 5.1   Lynn's story: the student as a change agent

After several years of working as a staff nurse in an intensive therapy unit (ITU), Lynn had successfully gained a place on the health visiting course. Lynn had worked hard over the last two years to develop an understanding of contemporary community practice and was looking forward to the course.

Two months later, Lynn started the course and over the first three weeks she was introduced to the programme and to her practice teacher, Joyce. Joyce was a very well organized practice teacher, and she had clearly mapped out the first few months of Lynn's placement. Lynn welcomed this structured approach, as the course was very intensive, with the first two assignments being due for submission within the first six weeks. Lynn's personal tutor, Hilda, explained how the dissertation required Lynn to identify a clinical practice development on which she would work over the duration of the course. She explained how the development should be small scale, and how Lynn would be required to plan, implement and evaluate the development in that period. Hilda said that Lynn would be required to select the specific area she wished to develop within the next two weeks, otherwise she would fall behind.

Lynn was anxious that here she was less than a month into the course and she was being asked to identify an area of practice she needed to change. To date, she had only completed eight practice placement days, and she felt that she had little understanding of the health visitor's role. Joyce said that she felt Lynn should look at weaning, as this was an interesting area of practice. Lynn reluctantly agreed, although at this time, she had little understanding of what this would involve.

During the remainder of the course Lynn worked to develop an information booklet on weaning for parents. She successfully managed to complete the course, but she found the production of her dissertation particularly difficult, because she had little interest in the topic area.

---

develop. As a result, Lynn was left to work on a development over which she had little ownership and for which the ground work had already been prepared by her practice teacher. Clearly, the degree of learning that will result from such a false situation will be negligible. The students will be left feeling that they simply have to follow instructions to pass the course, and not to attempt to follow anything too contentious.

In addition to the student, other people within this partnership suffer because of this approach. The student's practice teacher often experiences difficulties identifying a development that will not lead to increased workload for the practice team once the student has left. The nightmare situation would be for a practice teacher to have six additional specialist clinics to run, each one set up over successive years by students on a one-year placement.

These difficulties often lead to poorly planned, superficial developments that are not sustainable after the student has left. This raises a number of ethical issues about whether it is appropriate to establish a new service or aspect of care, if that service cannot be sustained in the longer term. Additionally, risk assessment is often compromised, because the student needs to implement a new development in such a short timescale.

In the last few years, nurse education has seen students studying for a first degree moving away from carrying out research. The rationale for this was that often the research was of a very poor quality, and did not lead to improvements in practice. It could be argued that practice development as part of higher education, for the purpose of teaching a student how to manage and lead change, is inappropriate. The inappropriateness of this approach assumes that the development of practice as part of a course is a straightforward method of demonstrating competence and theoretical understanding. However, the escalating complexities of health care delivery have made it more and more difficult for individuals to develop practice without the impact cascading across the organization.

Education has developed several specific approaches to the development of practice. Table 5.1 describes them, and also includes details of how these approaches are sometimes perceived by students and colleagues from the practice setting.

Issues of clinical credibility

If education is to play a role in promoting best practice, then its staff must be seen to be up to date and clinically credible. Nurse education's move into university has placed additional demands on teaching staff, which has put even greater pressure on some of the aspects of the nurse teacher's role, which in the past were seen as essential components of the role, for example placement links. In addition to contact time with students, clinical liaison and clinical credibility, academic staff are increasingly expected to participate in research and write for publication. Unlike medicine, we do not appear to have satisfactorily enabled nurses to continue clinical practice as well as teaching and researching, although others (Logue 1996) have called for teaching to be valued, and an end to the snobbery directed to those who teach by those who are able to both research and teach.

Various attempts have been made to try and bridge the divide between theory and practice, including clinical teachers, and more recently, the development of lecturer/practitioner roles (Lathlean 1997). Despite these attempts at maintaining and enhancing clinical credibility, the debate rages on about whether lecturers have to continue practising to maintain clinical credibility, or whether regular contact with the clinical areas is enough. Maybe the answer to this thorny issue lies in exploring lecturers'

Table 5.1 Bringing practice development into the educational arena

Strategies	Student's view	Practice view
Tripartite contracts	Students are placed in an unenviable position between at least two masters. Tutor and practice supervisor may have established relationship into which student enters. Alternatively, mutual ambivalence between academic tutor and practice supervisor may result in student needing to play mediator.	Contracts are elitist and place students in privileged position. The ability to replicate their changes in practice is unrealistic as students have protected time and have access within hierarchy via their supervisor.
Students as change agents	Puts student in an impossible situation – caught between pragmatics of getting through academic course and pressure of being seen to do well. Changes in practice attached to academic assessment add to student pressures as they need to be able to articulate processes as well as ensuring successful implementation of development.	Practice development seen as something only done when students are around. Innovations are delayed until the student is in place to see it through. Other practitioners don't feel they have time in 'everyday life'. Developments are not owned by all practitioners and are seen as time limited entities while student is in placement. Other practitioners see that ideas are given to student which makes them feel uninvolved and they have no sense of ownership.
Assessment of practice competence	Who does the assessment can be problematic as interpersonal relationships may colour competence in practice.	Difficulty in deciding what ought to be assessed within practice, and what methods should be used to assess competence within the clinical area. Patient/client safety should be paramount and risk assessment is now more important. Clinical practice not designed for the assessment of practice and patient/client care should not be compromised or manipulated to facilitate assessment.
Reflection	Onus on student to be able to come up with the goods and moves responsibility from teacher needing to know much about practice. Reflection is the province of students – lecturers facilitate, don't have to do it themselves.	Seen as a luxury activity that can only be indulged in during stints in education. Protestations are always about no time being available to do it in real life.

attitudes to the clinical environment, and whether they see themselves in a facilitating role, or whether they see themselves as the source of all knowledge and therefore need to know 'everything'.

The discussions about the theory–practice gap in nurse education may have been directed at educationalists not being in touch with the real world of nursing (Ferguson and Jinks 1994) but it could also be directed towards the clinical practitioners. Practitioners who attend educational sessions like empty vessels waiting to be filled with knowledge and skills from the teacher are likely to be very disappointed. Modern approaches to postregistration education rely upon practitioners sharing their knowledge with others as part of a two-way process, which educates both the nurse and the teacher. 'The teacher is no longer merely the one who teaches, but one who is himself [*sic*] taught in dialogue with the students, who in their turn, while being taught also teach' (Freire 1972: 53). The quotation from Freire encapsulates a specific approach to education, with the belief that the role a teacher should play in practitioners' learning is as a facilitator and enabler, and not as the fount of all knowledge.

Keeping up to date in nursing and health care practice poses a particular challenge to nurse educationalists. The pace of change in the health service, and the pressure that puts practitioners under, makes entering the clinical environment a minefield. The method of keeping up to date has to be reconsidered. Visiting students in their clinical placements does not necessarily achieve keeping up to date, nor does facilitating practice projects in higher degrees. We need to examine how we talk and write about practice, and then look at where the gaps between theory and practice are perceived to be. We have a lot to learn about the language we use, rather than just what people do! We also need to explore the idea of two-way traffic in education. Practice has a lot to teach education, and what we need to be able to do within education is to give practitioners skills and confidence in articulating what the issues in practice might be. 'Nursing has not been valued for its autonomous social contributions, independent decision making, scholarly productivity or collective striving for recognition, power, legitimisation in professional, political and policy making' (Reilly and Perrin 1999: 3).

Rogers and Freiberg (1994) advocate a humanistic approach to adult learning, one that values a positive relationship between teacher and learner. Coulter (1990) describes how applying humanistic approaches to nurse education can develop students into lifelong learners who are encouraged to continue to be self-directed in their learning both during their initial professional education, as well as afterwards. This process is in complete contrast to the approach that puts the teacher at the centre of the activity providing instruction (Rogers 1996). The teacher is regarded as a designer and manager of instruction and the sole evaluator of student learning. Behaviourist theories suggest that learning occurs when we receive outside stimuli and then respond (Rogers 1996). The teacher is seen as directing this process by the selection of stimuli and indicating to the student the approved response (Rogers 1996). This approach to teaching and learning stresses the active role of the teacher and the passive role of the student.

◯ Enabling practitioners to develop practice

Enabling through learning strategies

Those working in higher education should be developing practitioners and nurturing their quest for understanding and knowledge. A curious practitioner is one who will think about what they are doing within their practice, and the one who will want to develop and improve what they do with clients/patients. Nurturing practitioners requires a new approach to nurse education, where there is a move away from the behaviourist approach, which was largely teacher centred, towards a more humanistic student centred approach, which encourages the student to take responsibility for their own learning. This approach to learning has received a lot of criticism in recent years (Quinn 1995), as it does not acknowledge how human relationships and social contexts influence people's behaviour. However, proponents of this approach highlight that behaviourist theories underpin all theories of learning, and thus have a great deal of validity (Rogers 1996). This validity can be argued in terms of a stimulus–response model that, although the response might be different, learning still relies on a response to a stimulus, whether it is within a social context (humanistic theories) or from the demands of the subject matter (cognitive theories). The behaviourist approach to education has had a huge impact on nurse teaching and learning, and behaviours have been used to indicate levels of nursing practice (Benner 1984). Coulter (1990) has argued that there is still a place for a behaviourist approach to teaching and learning in nurse education, as skills acquisition is important in facilitating transitions into new roles and responsibilities.

Humanist approaches to nurse education, on the other hand, are seen to enshrine the values of higher education of the early twenty-first century. They also seek to rid nurse educators of the legacy of the traditional approach to nurse education (Hurst 1985). This traditional approach to nurse education was predicated on training rather than education. Nursing students were taught what tutors thought they needed to know, and they were expected to absorb facts and perform tasks blindly, without questioning the rationale for the information given to them (Burnard 1989). Many practitioners who trained as nurses before the late 1980s, experienced this kind of approach. Hurst (1985) has stated that this approach to nurse education concentrated on the medical model, such as learning anatomy and physiology, at the expense of higher order thinking, and centred on the status of the nurse teacher. The nurse teacher has the knowledge, and only allows access to this knowledge as and when they choose; there is no encouragement of self-discovery or creativity (Burnard 1989).

There is an implicit assumption that a programme of study that says it is student centred along with the use of reflective practice (Schön 1991) will meet student needs with little effort from teaching staff. Any deficiencies in the experience are the student's fault, as they have failed to respond and engage in the process of education. This approach fails to acknowledge the responsibilities of the teacher, who just simply turns up in the classroom and performs for the students. The beliefs of teaching staff do not appear to have been explored and consequently students witness a disparity between what they expect and what they are witnessing. There needs to be reciprocity between teacher and student, where the student feels valued and can engage in debate with the teacher in a safe and non-judgemental environment. If students are to grow and gain in confidence in the experience, surely teachers should be nurturing, rather than being critical and distant.

Being student centred means not being teacher centred, and this can be challenging and risky for the lecturer, who is used to being in control, both in the classroom and within tutorials (Rogers and Freiberg 1994). This adds a political dimension, as it requires a shift in power and control. If nursing is to become more empowered as a profession, then it appears that teachers of nursing will have to shift and re-examine their current approach, which often leaves much of the learning to the student (Harden 1996). Such approaches can add considerably to the stress levels of the student, which, in turn, have a significant impact on the learning of our students. The dissonance experienced by the students fuels this stress thus making the programme of study a very negative and disabling experience. If we are to encourage students to be lifelong learners, and be willing to engage in ongoing reflective practice, then there needs to be a reappraisal of the approach many take in their teaching practice. Reflection may not be the panacea that many consider it to be, but at least if practitioners consider their approach, then students may begin to have a positive and self-enhancing experience, and will be able to connect theory to practice.

Enabling through reflection

Reflective practice has become the mantra for nursing education in the late 1990s. As a response to the theory–practice gap, it is seen as both enabling nurses to make sense of the working world, as well as providing education with a legitimate toe-hold into practice (Rafferty *et al.*

1996). Although reflective practice is now becoming the new ortho-
doxy, few commentators have considered the implications, both in terms
of approaches to teaching, and the moral and ethical dimensions of
using practice situations within the classroom (Hargreaves 1997).

Reflection within nursing practice is seen as a way of empowering
nurses by enabling them to become aware of how they have come to
practice the way they have, by identifying the 'personal and professional
histories which shape their practice, the symbols and images inherent in
their language and the myths and metaphors which sustain them in
practice' (Street 1991: 1).

Although this approach is commendable, how reflective practice is
facilitated within education may be problematic, with the complexity of
all of the factors identified thus far. There may be many ways that some
teachers provide an environment in which students may readily identify
the sources of their oppression; other teachers may be oppressive and
hold positions of power that leave students marginalized and disillusioned. The concept of reflection, although eulogized by many commentators, lacks any clear definition, and thus is open to many interpretations
(Carr 1996; Mackintosh 1998; Taylor 2000). This then leads to teachers
developing their way of reflecting, and thus inculcating in students that
their way is the best and only way to reflect. This then leads to the
tyranny of having to be able to spot the right way to present your
reflections on your own work, and then be exposed to assessment of
these endeavours.

Reflection in action

Conway (1994) writes about how practitioners can use reflection in action
to create new knowledge and engage in this process in parallel with performance. The conditions for this activity to be identified as such should:

- occur in the practice setting;
- require the practitioner to think on her/his feet;
- involve a form of action research;
- cannot be taught but coaching can encourage its development;
- can be seen in the performance of practitioners who demonstrate
  'professional artistry';
- can be used as a paradigm case for learning from practice.

(Conway 1994: 114)

A number of writers have highlighted the problem with the definition
of reflective practice (James and Clarke 1994; Carr 1996; Mackintosh
1998). A lack of a definition has become problematic in terms of the
acceptance of the activity as a legitimate source of knowledge creation.
This is discussed at greater length in Chapter 2.

Supporting reflective practice

The certainty of adequate support mechanisms available in the practice setting to enable practitioners to cope with the tensions that rear their head when engaged in a critical enquiry of one's practice are questionable (Fitzgerald 1994). Many students on the undergraduate postregistration community degree have to manage a tripartite relationship between themselves, their practice supervisor and their personal tutor (educationalist). There could be occasions where the educationalist and practice supervisor have an established relationship, and appear to exclude the student from the meeting by talking about personal issues and shared past experiences. These behaviours by perceived role models only reinforce to the student their lowly and transitory status, and increase feelings of vulnerability and stress levels (see Isabel's story, Box 5.2).

As can be seen from Isabel's story, that experience affected both Isabel's attitude towards district nursing, but also may have profoundly influenced subsequent engagements with the development of practice. A negative experience like this is likely to discourage Isabel from taking any further initiatives in practice. Her relationship with both practice supervisor and tutor undermined her confidence and left her feeling that she was not worthy to take practice forward, as it is only done when you have successfully navigated secret rites of passage. This is a culture that should be actively discouraged, and adequate support systems for practice teachers should enable them to work with students in partnership with higher education, rather than colluding in an 'us and them' scenario.

◯ Professional developer

Higher education is well placed to encourage the development of practice through the provision of professional development programmes, which enhance the students' knowledge base and clinical skills within a particular aspect of clinical care. There is increasing pressure on NHS employers to enable practitioners to maintain continuing professional development (DoH 1998d). The introduction of the concept of clinical governance identifies lifelong learning and continuing professional development as pivotal to the development and maintenance of quality services within the health and social care (Swage 2000). This drive towards continuing professional development challenges nurse education to respond to the learning needs of the practice arena. This requires a different engagement with practice and will prove challenging to many who see themselves at the centre of the knowledge universe. Both educators and researchers will need to acknowledge that learning can take

---

Box 5.2 Isabel's story: the problems with tripartite contracts

Isabel is a part-time student on the community degree. She is an experienced community staff nurse, and has worked with the same district nursing team for some years. Her best friend is also a district nurse in a neighbouring trust. For her practice placement during the course, she has been allocated an experienced community practice teacher (CPT) in a different area of the trust. It soon becomes clear to Isabel that she is not going to get on very well with her CPT. There are evidently some strong feelings about the team that Isabel usually works with, and there are a number of comments made about how they do district nursing 'over there'. This makes Isabel feel very uncomfortable, but she feels that in her current position as a student she cannot comment, as she is reliant on the CPT to pass 50 per cent of the course, and does not want to get on the wrong side of her.

Isabel struggles with this dilemma, but as a pragmatist she feels that she can deal with the tensions, and it will provide plenty of material for her reflective diary. This was fine until the next meeting between her CPT and the university tutor. Isabel found the first meeting difficult, as she felt there were two agendas to the meeting. The first was about checking out her progress, and the second was about the two others in the relationship scoring points off each other. They had clearly known each other for a great deal of time, and had an uneasy alliance. They often excluded Isabel from the early part of the conversation as they caught up with the gossip within the trust, and talked about mutual acquaintances. This served to underline their familiarity with each other. This made Isabel feel very excluded, and she felt that her relationship with the CPT was further compromised by the ambiguous relationship between the CPT and the tutor. She felt that they were testing her out, rather than attempting to facilitate her learning and skills development.

Her first year report highlighted the problems in the relationship. The CPT had indicated that Isabel was not competent to progress on the course. Isabel was devastated by this assessment, and decided to make her concerns about roles and relationships known to her manager. Following this meeting, she was allocated a different CPT but still had the same tutor from the university. The following summer she successfully completed the degree programme, but this experience made her feel very bitter about the course. As a consequence, she decided not to be a district nurse anymore, and has obtained a post in a local hospice.

---

place within the practice setting, and that their role may be in optimizing the learning taking place, rather than being seen to be the source of knowledge. The challenge will be for higher education institutions to accept and accredit the learning that is taking place. This can be achieved in several ways, including Accreditation of Prior Experiential Learning (APEL) and Accreditation of Work Based Learning (AWBL).

Credit where credit's due

APEL and AWBL are both becoming increasingly important mechanisms in both encouraging lifelong learning and widening access to higher education. Both systems acknowledge that learning can take place outside the classroom, and that the traditional delivery mode of classroom teaching is not the only way that people gain knowledge. Just as Eraut (1994) has questioned the assumption that researchers are the source of all new knowledge, APEL questions whether all learning takes place when attending taught courses in educational institutions (Quinn 1995). AWBL, as a relatively new development, has received little critical attention to date. As Quinn (1995) has stated, there has been an assumption that the institutions of higher education know best, and alongside that assumption, the teachers and the content and type of learning that takes place is prescribed by the educational institution.

The recognition of APEL and AWBL has challenged this view, and in most pragmatic institutions there is an increasing acknowledgement that learning can take place in the practice setting, and that it is possible to award this learning academic currency. Of course not all experience leads to learning, but both APEL and AWBL require the participant to provide evidence of their learning, and thus requires them to examine what they have undertaken in practice, and articulate that learning to the satisfaction of academic bodies. APEL is always awarded retrospectively, and students normally seeking to gain admission onto a university course need to demonstrate the relevance of their experiential knowledge to the course they wish to undertake.

AWBL is prospective, and as such it has recently become a way of facilitating developments within practice that might have happened anyway. There have been murmurings that APEL (and probably AWBL, although because it is a fairly recent development it has been subjected to less discussion) systems dilute academic standards, and stand to jeopardize the professional status of nursing. However if mechanisms exist to ensure equivalence of learning between APEL, AWBL and traditional modes of learning, then the academic content should be rigorously assessed within all.

As can be seen within Judith's story (Box 5.3) the APEL mechanism facilitated access to an undergraduate programme, and clearly identified the learning and knowledge acquisition that took place during the development of practice. The learning that was identified within this project helped inform Judith's practice development activity within her degree studies. She was also able to compare the two experiences and explore the role of students in the development of practice. As a respected and experienced staff nurse, she was able to engage in the development without many problems, but as a student she encountered a number of

Box 5.3   Judith's story: using APEL to recognize practice development

Judith is an experienced community staff nurse who wishes to access the specialist practitioner degree. She currently has half the required number of academic credits for entry to the degree programme and knows she needs 120 to meet the academic entry criteria for the degree course. She has contacted the university about accreditation of experiential learning, as it appears to be the most appropriate and quickest way to gain the remaining number of academic credits. Her first meeting with the university tutor indicates the work involved, and although it appears rather daunting, as it is work related, should not be that difficult.

Judith has been working with the Macmillan nurse in her trust to provide better information about syringe drivers for patients and carers. She feels that although patients and carers are given permission to boost doses, and participate in symptom control, they are often reluctant to do so. She feels this is due to lack of information about how the syringe driver works and not fully understanding the drugs used in symptom management. The development Judith has in mind relates to patients and carers and what information they might like about syringe drivers. From this activity, she has developed a comprehensive leaflet that explains the use of the syringe driver, and advises patients and carers about basic problem solving, and also provides contact telephone numbers.

From the tutor's perspective, Judith has clearly worked very hard on her own initiative, and is keen that this development is recognized academically. The first step is to identify learning outcomes, and then encourage Judith to both articulate what she has learnt and also to demonstrate the evidence to support her involvement in the initiative.

In order for Judith to do this, she needs to present a portfolio that includes reflective writing and examples of the work she has done. The second meeting with the tutor helps to identify the most appropriate learning outcomes, and they then discuss what Judith should write about, and what evidence she ought to include in the portfolio.

This second meeting then launches Judith into the actual process of compiling the evidence and written work – this takes two months, and at the end of this, her tutor reviews the content and suggests Judith submit it for assessment and accreditation. Between them they agreed the following learning outcomes:

1 Identify clear rationale for development, and indicate process of consultation with patients, carers and colleagues.
2 Demonstrate knowledge of the different and complementary roles of each discipline in the support of patients and carers.
3 Discuss own role in facilitating the development of practice and articulate the steps taken in the process of development.

Following successful submission of her portfolio, Judith went on to study in the degree course, where she obtained a 2:1 degree and has continued to be involved in developing practice as district nursing sister.

obstacles, the most important of these being the time available for the development. Educational imperatives constrain developments as a result of both the time available for the course and artificial timescales.

Finally, all of the educational approaches that can support the development of practice are dependent upon the practitioner having the skills and competence to be able to lead and manage change. The drive towards competence-based learning outcomes in higher education has gone some way to ensuring that practitioners feel prepared to meet these challenges. As part of the drive to become recognized as a profession, the theoretical basis of nursing has been promoted at the expense of the realities of practice. This has led to the criticism from some quarters that nurses are not being adequately prepared for practice.

In order to counter this argument, there needs to be a radical rethink about what the learning outcomes of a programme of study should be, and how and by whom they should be assessed. At present, there is a greater emphasis on the academic level of work that often threatens and challenges experienced practitioners, as they feel undermined by the expectations. Students supervised by senior practitioners often experience a conflict about the competence base of the course requirements (assessed by a practice teacher) and the academic rigour demanded by university tutors. There is often a mismatch, and criticism is often aimed at the practitioners and blame placed on them for not accessing professional development. In order to supervise students adequately on the new breed of academic courses, practice teachers should be provided with a comprehensive support package that couples information about course requirements and ensures their continuing competence to supervise students. This should be provided as a part of the continuing professional development offered to other university assessors within the institutions of higher education. If we are working in partnership, then we should treat practice supervisors/assessors with the respect that they deserve – surely this would enhance the culture of lifelong learning in the health service? This partnership would also help all interested parties to define and agree upon those competencies they wish students to achieve and also agree how they are best assessed.

Box 5.4 provides a very positive example of higher education. A competence-based approach not only has a developmental effect on the individual, but also has an impact on the working environment. The competence model encouraged Maureen to examine the impact of acquiring new skills on the team within which she worked. It also created a dialogue between herself and others within the practice. This might not have happened if the skills were developed in a singular role development. By critically examining the process of skill development, it has enabled Maureen to legitimately examine parallel practice developments by her colleague. This has encouraged mutual learning that has greatly

---

Box 5.4   Maureen's story: using education to facilitate the development of practice

Maureen is an experienced community nurse who has recently completed a community degree and qualified as a health visitor. Over the last two years, she has become increasingly aware that during the routine baby clinic, parents are presenting with a number of queries that, as a practice nurse, she might have addressed, but are outside the immediate remit of her health visitor role. These queries include rashes, coughs and colds etc. It appears that parents are reluctant to access the GP, and see the baby clinic as an ideal opportunity to ask about things that are worrying them, either about their child or themselves. They become quite frustrated that they then have to make a further appointment to see the GP or practice nurse. This not only frustrates the parents, it also frustrates Maureen who felt that her previous clinical experience, combined with additional skills development, would equip her to provide a more comprehensive service.

Following discussion with her manager and the GPs in the practice, it is agreed that she can attend a course that combines clinical skills development with exploring the implications of an expanded nursing role. The course content includes history taking, clinical examination techniques and ordering of appropriate tests. It is a competence-based course that expects the student to critically reflect on the process of skills development, as well as the outcomes at the end of the course.

Maureen has a personal tutor from the university, a nurse mentor and a GP supervisor to support her in a tripartite contract. At the beginning of the course, it becomes evident that one of her practice nurse colleagues is going to attend a nurse practitioner course, and this highlights some tensions within the practice about role demarcation and resource negotiations (particularly over which GP is going to provide mentorship). However, instead of this becoming a barrier to relationship development, it proves to be a catalyst for increasing communication within the team, and an acknowledgement that each practitioner can contribute different services for different client groups.

Maureen felt that if she had just tried to implement the development of her role without the educational framework, she would have become unstuck once the initial conflict was highlighted. However because the course provided very different frameworks for the students to work with, then this clearly identified to the practice team that there was room for both practitioners to develop their role. Agreeing that the role developments were complementary rather than conflicting enabled not only a better service for patients, but also a better working relationship within the team.

improved their working relationship. This might not always happen, but if done sensitively and purposefully, may go a long way to facilitate better working relationships within any team. It would be wonderful to see that when practitioners engage in educational activity, they also enhance their working environment.

◯ Conclusion

As can be seen, the relationship between the development of practice and education is not an easy or simple one. Both need each other, but instead of a parasitic relationship, there should be a symbiotic relationship, where both grow from each other. There needs to be mutual respect, but this can only be achieved if it is deserved. Practitioners need to demonstrate responsiveness to patient/client need, and recognition that ritualistic routinized practice, although a good safety valve, might be counter-productive to both job satisfaction and patient/client well-being. Alongside this, education needs to recognize the value of clinical practice, and seek to help practitioners understand their work, rather than undermine it by labelling it as 'not of sufficient academic rigour'. A creative dialogue needs to happen between practice and education to enable each to understand and to value each other. This can happen if the educational experience is positive and enhancing. Education staff should encourage student ability and nurture talent. This is not easy and cannot happen overnight, but the relationship between education and practice can be improved using a common language that all can understand.

More flexible approaches to learning, such as APEL and AWBL, will enable practitioners to articulate the learning that takes place within the practice setting. It will also lead to recognition of the cognitive skills they have developed as a consequence of developing their practice. This will help to create a more equal relationship between practice and education, and dispel the theory–practice gap debate. Developing practice is never easy or straightforward. However, the engagement with education within that process should not hinder or inhibit practitioners' enthusiasm for improving patient/client experiences. Educational experiences should provide a platform for practitioners to take ideas forward within their practice. The provision of this platform to practitioners will give them added confidence that they are doing the right thing. Being able to identify the evidence that underpins the development alongside knowledge of the theoretical concepts that provide insight into facilitating the process of developments will ensure that developments in practice are successful and sustainable.

Part (III) Key issues when developing practice

6 Can you feel the force? The importance of power in practice development

Wendy Burke

◯ Chapter summary

In this chapter some short case studies are presented, which provide examples of practice development in four of the community nursing specialisms. After each case study, the key themes that emerge are explored in detail, and strategies that can help practitioner's work through issues raised are identified. Readers are strongly advised not to be tempted to read only the case study that relates to their specific specialism, but to explore each one. The themes – namely conflict, primary to secondary care shift, medical dominance, negotiation and user perspectives – that emerge from the case studies are of relevance to nursing practice development generally.

◯ Case study 1: 'fight the good fight'

'Bloody tribalism!' screamed Fiona as she replaced the telephone handset. She had just received another irate call from a local school nurse, Cynthia Hardwick, to enquire why she was seeing Claire Graham, a 7-year-old with cerebral palsy. Cynthia had accused her of undermining Claire's mother's confidence in the school health service by taking over her care and starting treatment for her daytime incontinence problems. Cynthia was one of a long line of school nurses and health visitors who were going to complain to their manager, Miss Arlington, about the role of the community children's nurse, and in particular, about Fiona.

Fiona wondered why she had bothered to take the job in the first place. As she boiled the kettle, she quietly seethed about the constant criticism levelled at her by her colleagues from the community trust. If only there were more community children's nurses in the trust, Fiona would not feel so isolated; as it was, she simply 'chewed over' the issues by herself. She felt that one of the reasons why there was so much animosity about her work, was that she was employed by the acute trust, while the majority of her work involved contact with people from primary care.

Fiona wondered why she had bothered to develop new services when it caused such aggravation. Her mind jumped to the past bad experiences since she had commenced her specialist continence service for children with special needs. Just as quickly, she started remembering some of her great successes, and the feelings she had when she managed to relieve some of the obvious burden on parents and other carers, as the children achieved continence. Her mood lightened as she realized that she was in the right and the others were in the wrong.

Suddenly Fiona was startled by a loud knock at her office door. It was her manager Sandy, who had called to see her after receiving a telephone call from Miss Arlington. This was the third complaint against Fiona since she started her specialist clinic nine months ago, but in her own mind, this was more serious because in four weeks' time both the acute and community trusts were merging to form a combined trust.

Sandy flopped down into the chair and kicked off her shoes. 'Get me a cuppa, Fiona luv', remarked Sandy. Fiona duly obliged and they both sat back for a chat. Sandy told Fiona about the call and laughed about the fact that Miss Arlington had nothing better to do than ring up and complain that she should ring every Tom, Dick and Harry to keep them informed about who she was seeing. Fiona was relieved that Sandy was so supportive of her work and her role. She was, however, concerned about whether things would be quite so supportive after the merger.

Half an hour later, Fiona was in out-patients, running her busy continence clinic. She had a student community children's nurse with her today from the local university. Fiona told the student that when she first started in her role, she was struck by the sheer number of children with bladder problems. Some children were lucky enough to get expert advice and help from the paediatricians, and some school nurses and health visitors had special interest in the field, and were very supportive. Other children received no help and parents struggled with toilet training programmes, often with frustrating consequences and ultimate failure. Fiona explained that sometimes achieving continence in children with disabilities was really easy. Often parents were reluctant to start toilet training, because they had low expectations about the child ever achieving dryness, or the parents left the child in nappies or pads because it was easier. 'Don't get me wrong', explained Fiona, 'I don't blame parents for not trying training programmes. They've got so much else to contend with, that they need a lot of support to even begin to try.'

Fiona decided to set up the special clinic almost a year ago, and it had now been running for nine months. At the time, she discussed it with her consultant colleagues and her manager. With hindsight, she acknowledged that it would have been sensible to have shared her plans with staff from the community trust. Indeed, on many occasions, she could do with support from people like the community learning disabilities team. But there was no going back now, the damage was done. Now she was only a few weeks away from working with the same staff she had obviously upset.

Four months later, Fiona felt physically sick at the thought of attending her first team meeting in the new Child Health Directorate. The directorate was part of the new combined trust, and encompassed paediatrics, community children's nursing, health visiting and school nursing. The directorate was managed at the moment by Kathleen, a former health visitor, who so far had been very supportive of the work of community children's nurses. At two o'clock, Fiona arrived at the meeting and opened the door with trepidation. As she walked into the room, she spotted Mandy, a school nurse who had attended university at the same time as herself. She sat with Mandy and caught up with her news. Fiona told Mandy about her problems over the last few months since she had set up her specialist clinic. Mandy said that she heard all about her work, and she told Fiona that not everyone was against her, indeed, several people would quite like to work with her to develop the service further.

The meeting passed quickly and at the end, Mandy introduced Fiona to several colleagues, who were interested in continence. She was surprised to learn that several school nurses already ran enuresis clinics, and Claire, a dynamic health visitor, was something of a specialist in childhood encopresis. The group decided that it would be really useful to meet up to talk about strategy, and plan a more coordinated approach. Fiona left the meeting and headed to her car in the car park. Driving back to the hospital, Fiona was amazed at how well the meeting had gone. She thought to herself that perhaps she had developed the wrong impression about the other professional groups, and indeed, she herself might have been guilty of a little 'professional tribalism' in the past.

Over the next few months, the team met regularly to look at the services they already had, and how the groups could work together to develop comprehensive continence services for all children. The group decided that a central referral system should be set up for all children with continence problems, and that the professionals involved should meet weekly to allocate cases on the basis of specialist skills. This new system worked very well and was liked by both GPs and consultants, because they no longer needed to ring around to see who the best person would be to see a particular child.

The new children's continence group was successful in achieving funding for equipment such as enuresis alarms through the local primary care group, who were heartened by the joint primary/secondary care approach to service delivery. Fiona could not help thinking how far they had come from petty squabbles about who should do what to something approaching a coordinated approach to care delivery.

Fiona continued her weekly clinic, but she now saw a much wider range of children with bladder and bowel problems. Her clinic had been much improved by the presence of Claire, a health visitor, because up until this point, Fiona had often been stumped when presented with bowel problems in children.

This case study clearly demonstrates the importance of managing conflict when leading change. Conflict arises whenever interests collide. It is defined by Marquis and Huston (1996: 333) as 'the internal discord that results from differences in ideas, values, or feelings between two or more people'. Johnson (1994) adds that conflict is created when there are differences in economic and professional values, and when there is competition among professionals. This was reflected in the case study as the tribalism that was witnessed from the health visitors and also admittedly by Fiona herself. Tribal ties lock individuals into a particular way of behaving and thinking about others who do not belong to their particular professional group. This behaviour leads to poor understanding of others' roles, mistrust and hostility, and as John Unsworth pointed out in Chapter 1, 'mars the working relationships' between groups of nurses, which could potentially create artificial barriers for patients.

The other source of conflict in this case study was due to poor communication. Conflict is inevitable if all participants do not have the same information. Any effective change process requires clear and consistent communication to all participants and influential parties. Lancaster (1999: 213) argues that 'it is not enough just to discuss the proposed plan with the anticipated participants'; everyone who could be affected by change needs to be informed and involved. Fiona admitted to herself that with hindsight she should have discussed the proposals with health visiting colleagues at a much earlier stage in developing the project.

The natural reaction to conflict is to view it as a dysfunctional force, as an unfortunate state that in more favourable circumstances would disappear, and comments such as 'It's a personality problem' and 'They're rivals who always meet head-on' are common statements that reflect this fact. It is, however, important to acknowledge that the clash, disagreement, or different perspectives that conflict brings can be viewed as both useful and a hindrance (Lancaster 1999). For example, in this particular case study, conflict was a negative force; it was disruptive for both Fiona and her health visiting colleagues, and it caused anger and wasted time in the complaints that were generated. Yet in some situations the expression of conflict can actually be constructive; it can encourage self-evaluation and challenge conventional wisdom, and while it may cause a certain degree of pain, it can also do much to stimulate learning and change (Morgan 1997). Conflict therefore may prevent stagnation and can be used as a tool for responding to and implementing change.

What is clearly demonstrated in the case study however, is that glossing over or ignoring conflict leaves the problem unsolved and can lead to further problems later. Accepting that conflict is a signal that something is amiss should generate action. The optimal goal in resolving conflict is creating a win–win solution for those involved. Realistically, this may not be possible in every situation, and perhaps the goal should be to lessen the perceptual differences that exist between parties. There are five common conflict resolution strategies (Morgan 1997: 206):

- compromising;
- competing;
- cooperating – accommodating – smoothing;
- avoiding;
- collaborating.

The choice of strategy will depend on the situation, the urgency, the importance of the issue, and so on. In the case study the conflict was avoided initially, until Fiona found herself in a position where she had to deal with it. The trusts were merging and she was going to be working in the same directorate as her health visiting colleagues.

For Fiona, the organizational climate was a factor in determining her response at this point in time. Organization climate, which is also referred to as culture, is like the weather. Changes in the weather indicate what is reasonable to wear or possible to do on any given day. The weather affects our relationships with others, and people treat one another quite differently on a clear, bright summer's day versus a stormy grey day. Organizational climate similarly affects the behaviour and interactions of people. While organizational climate is not something that we can directly see, it can however be perceived and sensed.

While Fiona could distance herself from the conflict in the short term, she was very aware that her position could be severely compromised in the future, when the trusts merged. She needed a win–win solution. Fiona used collaboration, a cooperative means of resolving conflict. She was able, with some of her health visiting colleagues, to work together, breaking down some of those tribal ties so that both sides could offer a perspective to identify problems and search for the most effective solution. The focus then was on solving problems and not necessarily on winning at all costs.

Johnson (1994) maintains that collaboration is the best method to resolve conflict to achieve long-term benefit. It can however be a lengthy process. Langford (1981: 113) describes the following steps as key in the process:

1 define a common goal on which both parties can agree;
2 mutually respect the knowledge and expertise of all parties;
3 work together to review the goal once it is reached;
4 communicate honestly and openly;
5 have equitable, shared decision making powers;
6 share knowledge;
7 offer support;
8 understand the language and terms inherent;
9 have mutually acceptable roles.

In conclusion, the most common source of conflict is a communication problem, and any person seeking to influence or bring about change must recognize and understand the factors that facilitate the communication process, as well as the commonly occurring obstacles.

○ Case study 2: 'shifting the load'

Nancye had been feeling for some time now that there had to be more to life as a practice nurse in a busy GP practice than cervical smears and taking blood. It wasn't that she was dissatisfied, but she knew she was capable of more. She just needed the right opportunity. It came sooner than she thought, and it began simply by an increasing awareness that the number of patients discharged from hospital who were being prescribed warfarin and required INR (International Normalized Ratio) monitoring was rapidly increasing. These patients were fast becoming a growing problem in the practice, because there was no service to meet their needs as they had traditionally been managed within the hospital setting.

In order for patients to have their INR monitored, and ensure that they were taking the correct dose of warfarin, they had to make an appointment with the practice nurse to have a blood specimen taken. This was for many patients a weekly appointment. They were told to ring the reception staff two days later for the result of the test. The laboratory results were filed on a daily basis within the practice for each GP to look at. On the basis of the results, GPs were required make any necessary changes in the warfarin dose.

Patients were anxious for their results, and they would often have to ring the practice on numerous occasions because of the difficulties associated with reception staff chasing up GPs who had often not had the opportunity to look at the laboratory results. In addition, most GPs had little knowledge of or interest in anticoagulation management, which had been in the past predominantly secondary care led. So there was a growing problem in the practice and a daily occurrence of irate and dissatisfied patients and reception staff, who did not enjoy playing 'piggy in the middle', bearing the brunt of both GPs' and patients' frustrations.

Another problem was that some patients chose to go to the local district general hospital, some eight miles away, to have their INR monitored because it provided a one-stop shop. Blood test, results and review of warfarin dose were carried out at one visit. However, this clinic was very impersonal and patients often endured a wait of half a day – almost longer than you would expect to wait in A&E with a minor injury. In addition, the hospital clinic was always very busy. It was often standing room only – tiring and difficult, lost time for those in work, and almost impossible for the elderly or mothers with babies and young children. Not surprisingly, the patients complained bitterly about this service.

The situation then:

- increasing numbers of patients discharged from hospital on warfarin therapy;
- increasing numbers of patients requesting INR monitoring at the surgery as opposed to the hospital;
- no formalized procedure in the practice to deal with these patients;
- no identified staff trained to manage anticoagulation;
- poorly controlled patients (often less than 50 per cent of patients with their INR within recommended therapeutic range);
- a poorly managed and underdeveloped area within primary care.

Nancye saw the opportunity and grasped it. She began by sitting down with a vaguely interested GP and the head receptionist to discuss the issues. She made some suggestions, some small changes that might make life easier for everyone. The first suggestion was to create a specific clinic for these patients to have their blood taken in the practice on a specific day of the week. For those patients who were housebound, the auxiliary nurses who were part of the district nursing team agreed to visit and take their blood specimens on the same day that the clinic took place. All the lab results and patients' telephone calls for results were channelled directly to Nancye. Nancye and the GP (in consultation with the haematologist) wrote a protocol to manage these patients, including altering dosage if a patient's INR was outside their therapeutic range. Nancye spent hours ploughing through medical records in the practice, ensuring that all patients had an identified therapeutic INR range written on their records, and where this was not available, she encouraged the GP to contact the haematologist at the local district general hospital. This was by far the most onerous task.

Nancye's learning curve was very steep. She spent hours in the library reviewing articles about warfarin management, time at the hospital pathology laboratory, and time at the hospital-based clinic, which was run largely by pharmacists. Within six months, her knowledge base had expanded, the patients were more satisfied, the GPs were delighted because no one bothered them, and the reception staff were ecstatic because it was one less thing to chase up the doctor for.

Nancye, however, felt that she had just scratched the surface, solving some of the initial problems but uncovering a plethora of other problems and she still felt frustrated. Why?

- Patients had little or no understanding of how warfarin worked, and the lifestyle issues that affected the therapeutic use. They simply had their blood taken and took the tablets as instructed.
- Taking venous blood and waiting a day for their result was, for some patients, a lot of hassle. Many patients worked – they hated the hospital, but going there got it over and done with in one visit. What the patients really wanted was a one-stop shop at the practice, without the long wait they endured at the hospital.
- GPs were delighted that Nancye had taken almost full responsibility for the management of these patients, but their withdrawal left her feeling totally unsupported.

So the journey continued. Nancye applied for funding through a Department of Health scholarship which was advertised in one of the nursing journals and, as a novice applicant, could not believe it when she was successful. This really spurred her on and gave her confidence in what she was doing. Nancye was able to resolve most of the outstanding problems.

She purchased 'near patient testing' equipment and computerized decision support software and created a database of all patients, so she was able to monitor how well controlled patients were within their therapeutic range. The clinic was redesigned, creating early appointments for patients to attend before work. The patients welcomed the changes and numbers grew steadily, removing the need for patients to travel out of the way to the hospital and endure long waits.

The whole experience of developing this area of practice was not without its problems. As Nancye's knowledge increased and her confidence steadily grew, the GPs continued to withdraw. They became increasingly unsure of how to relate to the new breed of nurse who, by their own admission, had more knowledge about anticoagulation management than they did. Nancye felt completely unsupported. However her response was to create other networks of support. She began by contacting the haematologist directly and asking for his opinion about certain patients who were more difficult to manage. He replied to her letters, but directed his correspondence directly to the patients' GP and completely bypassed her. This did not deter her. She persevered and continued to contact him, both in writing and by telephone. Initially, he was very rude and arrogant, then it suddenly occurred to Nancye that he might perceive her nursing development to be a threat, and also competition to the service delivered at the hospital. She continued to maintain regular contact with him, even referring patients to him directly, and as time went by, she managed to establish a solid working relationship with him based on mutual respect and understanding.

Similarly, there were ongoing problems of patients being discharged from hospital with no record of the last INR, target INR or dose of warfarin. Communicating with hospital consultants or junior doctors and being taken seriously as a nurse with considerable expertise in this field, without the support of the GP, was also initially very difficult. Yet today the haematologist remains Nancye's main source of advice and support. Her networks are now extensive, both locally and nationally, but she struggled to establish them as a nurse in what is predominantly a medical field.

The aim of anticoagulation therapy is to reduce the risk of a thrombo-embolic event, or the extension of an existing event, by maintaining patients at an optimal level of anticoagulation, without producing an unacceptable risk of haemorrhage. This balance is maintained by regular blood monitoring of their International Normalized Ratio (INR), which may then require alteration to their therapy. Nationally, anticoagulation therapy remains a poorly managed area within the NHS, largely because of its high-risk benefit, and the concomitant client-specific character-istics (Ansell 1998). Acute hospitals are unable to manage the increasing 20 per cent of patients each year being commenced on anticoagulation therapy. The majority of patients are on warfarin for life. They are very often active people, working and involved in their family life, and spend time on weekly to two monthly clinic visits for blood monitoring.

More of this work is being shifted to primary care because of the in-creasing numbers, the lack of capacity within acute hospitals to provide accessible and responsive services, and patient expectations of increased range of services in primary care. Like other speciality areas of practice traditionally managed by the secondary care sector, this shift is often happening without the resources or expertise to support it, and despite the enormous potential for medical fatalities.

The secondary to primary care shift was the main impetus for the development in this case study, and was an opportunity that Nancye was able to grasp. The interface between primary and secondary care has become a major focus of health policy debate. Primary care is cur-rently centre stage in the NHS plans for the future of health care in the

UK. Government policy to shift the balance and establish a primary care-led NHS has occurred in the face of rising consumer expectations, developing technologies and an ageing population. Rationalization of the secondary care sector into fewer and more specialized acute units, and the emergence of extended primary care organizations in the form of PCTs, means that there are increasing numbers of patients whose dependency and specialized needs previously may have indicated in-patient stay, but are now being cared for at home. Primary care provides the first contact to the great majority of health problems presented to the NHS and, together with the special features of primary care, which are deemed to be good and widely admired in other countries, provide the rationale behind moving to a primary care-led NHS. The special features of primary care – easy access, acceptability, person centred, comprehensive services, continuity, longitudinality (providing care over a long period) – maximize the overall aims of the health service. However within this setting, care is provided by generalists rather than specialists. The specialist has a narrow range of problem-specific skills, where in contrast the generalist has a broad range of competencies suited to dealing with both well-defined and undifferentiated problems.

The biggest single challenge to a primary care-led NHS is to maintain quality of care previously delivered by specialists in secondary care, and to build the capacity and expertise in meeting these needs within primary care. This case study clearly demonstrates such a challenge.

The smooth transition between the secondary and primary care interface is also essential. The challenges are: overcoming traditional boundaries and financial barriers caused by separate budgets, and helping some individual practitioners relinquish the power that they have been used to exercising. The case study identifies that collaboration at the interface is crucial, particularly when there are complex patient problems. Effective communication, in terms of sharing both knowledge and expertise, is the key. Practitioners from both sectors are dependent on each other for task definition and completion, as continuity of care cannot be achieved without the involvement of both. Abrupt transition to primary care, with the corresponding lack of communication identified in this case study, is not the ideal journey for patients. Attitudes and the practices of health care professionals, together with a new philosophy of cross boundary cooperation and negotiation at all levels, is increasingly important.

The increase in volume and ranges of services demanded of primary care and the decline in recruitment of some members of primary health care teams, notably GPs, have resulted in the need for expansion in the numbers and types of staff working within primary care and the development of new professional roles. Nowhere is this more visible than in community nursing. Nurse practitioners, specialist nurses and nurse consultants are examples of roles that require new independence and expertise. More community nurses, who are more assertive, educated and competent than ever before, are needed, like the new breed of nurse described in this case study, who grasped an opportunity to use her skills fully, and develop and extend her clinical role. However Nancye readily became a threat to doctors who were unaccustomed to being challenged, having professionally dominated the industry and division of labour for decades. Salvage and Smith (2000: 1019) state;

> The relationship between doctors and nurses has never been straight-forward. The differences of power, perspective, education, pay, status, class and, perhaps above all, gender have led to tribal warfare as often as peaceful co-existence. Nurses' readiness to be slighted, and doctors' reluctance to be challenged, create an undercurrent of tension. This may be masked in practice setting by the pressing need to get the work done, but it is there.

There are some who now believe that medicine is changing, perhaps reluctantly and by political expediency. Together with the changes in nursing, this is having a positive impact upon relationships. There are also broader societal changes, for example women are increasingly powerful in most sectors, and the medical profession now includes more women at every level. This offers great potential for relationships and practice. It undermines that traditional equation of female sex with low status.

Salvage and Smith (2000) believe that the time has come for doctors and nurses to let go of the resentments, an end to situations where an opportunity for one becomes a threat for the other. They suggest much more collaborative and cooperative approaches in order to leave the lingering traditional images of their professions behind.

> Instead of the boundary disputes and substitution squabbles, effort could be directed towards capitalising on the wealth of skills that all professionals can bring to bear on solving health problems. This fresh approach to the division of labour puts the patient at the centre for the first time.
>
> (Salvage and Smith 2000: 1020)

As the case study demonstrates, this may not be easy to achieve. Working in partnership takes time and effort, particularly where there are barriers to overcome. Effective partnerships based on equality, mutual trust and respect take time to establish in the context of a troubled past. Community nurses need to understand the tensions in the relationships between themselves and medical colleagues when developing practice and find ways, as Nancye did, to influence a positive outcome that will benefit patients.

◯ Case study 3: 'I've got the power'

Carole came back to the office looking gloomy, after another session with the headteacher in the local high school, firmly put in her place by the matronly Mrs Jakes, and told in no uncertain terms that she was 'only the school nurse' and 'any changes to do with sex education in this school would have to be put to the governors' and she simply didn't have time to discuss trivial issues. Mrs Jakes never seemed to have time for Carole. She felt her role as school nurse was not understood. She was always dismissed, put firmly in her place by the most senior person in the school, and she had never been given a real opportunity to present and thoroughly discuss her ideas. Carole was acutely aware that there was a myriad of problems in the school. It served a deprived area and faced above average truancy rates, drug and alcohol problems and high teenage pregnancy rates. Carole felt that she was an important member of the school team, and had a valuable part to play, yet she was really struggling to establish a role that was valued and respected by the head. There was never a room for her, yet she visited the school tirelessly on the same days every week. In fact, if she had a dedicated room, she could start up a drop-in session every day; she knew there was a need for it. Carole had lots of innovative ideas, and she also had a string of qualifications and lots of experience – teaching certificate, health promotion and family planning certificate. She was determined to use them for the benefit of pupils in that school.

Carole was very aware of the powerful position that Mrs Jakes played within the school. She ruled with a rod of iron, but was well liked and respected by her teaching staff. Carole knew that the head of guidance had recently retired on the grounds of ill health, and by pure chance overheard that Mr Crow had been appointed to the post. The rumour machine led Carole to believe he was a very different animal to most of the other teachers in the school. She saw a glimmer of hope. Immediately, she made an appointment to see him. Perhaps she might find an ally with whom she could really work.

Mr Crow was young and dynamic. He gave Carole a very enthusiastic welcome, and explained that he was delighted to meet her, as he had worked very closely with school nursing colleagues at his last school, and he had found them to be a very valuable resource. Carole outlined her concerns around the issues of the growing teenage pregnancy rate, lack of local health services for young people in the town, a sex education programme that didn't seem to be meeting the needs of pupils, and the historical difficulty in negotiating her role with the head.

Hallelujah! Mr Crow was eager to work with Carole on the issues she had raised. Over a period of two months, they began identifying key stakeholders who shared their views and ideas. A group was formed which defined the local problems and began to develop innovative solutions. The group was multiagency in nature, and included the manager of the sexual health service in the local community trust, the manager of the sexual health education team from the local education authority, the manager of the youth worker team and the health authority lead person for the Sexual Health Health Improvement Programme (HImP).

The group made the following recommendations:

- to provide joint training for the schoolteachers and school nurse in order to implement effective delivery of sex and relationship education;
- to provide a new sex and relationship programme in the school with dedicated teaching time for the school nurse. The programme they intended to use had emerged from a detailed review by the group of education programmes, both locally and nationally. The programme was underpinned by sound research and robust evaluation, and included a focus on the wider determinants of sexual behaviour in young people, examining self-esteem, relationships and life goals and not just the routine nuts and bolts of sexual intercourse;
- to provide a school nurse drop-in session every lunchtime, operating from a specific room in the youth block. Carole had been able to identify the need for this, by conducting some simple questionnaires with pupils in the school;
- to develop a young persons' community family planning clinic run by two youth workers, a family planning doctor and a family planning nurse. It was proposed that the clinic be provided in the nearby local community clinic, and held after school, once per week. Utilizing the evidence of other schemes for young people and demonstrating that young people were not accessing mainstream family planning services locally, the group proposed submitting a bid to a Sexual Health Health Improvement Plan Group for the next round of funding in order to develop this service.

The difficult task ahead was to convince the headteacher and the governors of their recommendations. Carole's past track record with the head had not been good. Mrs Jakes appeared to relish her powerful position as the head of the school. Access to the governors had always been denied and Mrs Jakes, in this gatekeeping role, had always given the impression that the governing body didn't like change. Mr Crow and Carole arranged to see the head. She had been kept informed of the progress of the working group by updates from Mr Crow and minutes of meetings.

Armed with the recommendations from the group, and supported by the latest report from the Social Exclusion Unit (Social Exclusion Unit 1999) and up-to-date information from the Teenage Pregnancy Unit, the local teenage pregnancy figures, and results of the questionnaire she had distributed, Carole felt as prepared as she could be. The reception from the headteacher was initially rather frosty. However she seemed to have a clear understanding of the issues, having kept track of the work of the group, and she appeared genuinely impressed at the amount of work and the collaborative networks established. Carole appeared calm and very self-assured throughout the meeting, and was able to demonstrate her considerable knowledge of the subject under discussion.

The suggestion that implementing the proposals from the group would establish the school as a beacon was particularly attractive to Mrs Jakes, together with the reassurance that her role was key in further developing and implementing the proposals. Mrs Jakes actually made the suggestion that the proposals should be put forward to the next meeting of the school governors, and Carole and Mr Crow were invited to present the proposals. Carole was delighted – what a breakthrough! The governors seemed pleased to receive the proposals. There was constructive debate and discussion and, while there were real concerns raised about some of the proposals, Mr Crow and Carole were able to provide adequate answers and reassurance. What appeared to convince the governors was the fact that Mrs Jakes was extremely supportive, and the governors voted unanimously in favour of implementing the proposals. Carole felt like she had lost an enemy and found a friend.

This case study demonstrates the importance of understanding the concept of power in implementing developments in practice, and how to become a successful negotiator. Power is present throughout every organization. It is typically feared and a source of concern. Nurses leading or effecting change need to understand the nature of power and its effective use, as well as its manipulative or abusive use. Some view power as a resource, as something one possesses, while others view it as a social relationship, characterized by some kind of dependency – as an influence over something or someone. In organizational terms, most take their point of departure from the definition of power offered by American political scientist Robert Dahl (1957), who suggests that power is the ability to require others to act as the power holder desires in a way that they would not otherwise have done. It is the strongest possible form of influence as people who wield it are often in positions to exert consequences that will have an effect on others. Power influences who gets what, when and how. It is the capacity to make or prevent things happening. In this case study, Mrs Jakes demonstrated her capacity as headteacher to prevent any changes that the school nurse suggested.

Power comes from a number of rich and varied sources (Morgan 1997). Lancaster (1999) describes the five main types. *Legitimate* or *position power* is power that is determined by designated authority in a role, position or office that is recognized and accepted by others. This is the most obvious source of power in an organization; position is defined in terms of rights and obligations, which create a field of influence and within which the person can legitimately operate. *Expert power* is based on the knowledge, skills or expertise of a person. It is related to information and the access to valued and desired information. Knowledge and information are a means of legitimizing what one wishes to do. Also often the expert carries an aura of authority. *Reward power* is based on offering inducements or positive sanctions. *Coercive power* is the opposite to reward power, based on negative sanctions or penalties, often based on fear of punishment or withholding rewards. *Referent power* is based on respect and admiration associated with charisma or the personal charm of the person.

In this case study, there are examples of two sources of power. First, Mrs Jakes demonstrates the use of legitimate or position power. As the headteacher, she has the authority accepted and recognized by others that allows her to make decisions and take responsibility for the running of the school. Mrs Jakes is in a dominant position, and she has a gatekeeping role. She has the power to make decisions that prevent changes from happening. While the decision making may be flawed, for example based on a lack of understanding or a personal dislike, or simply not be seen as high priority, nonetheless Mrs Jakes is in a position to make those decisions, and takes full responsibility for them. The second source of power is that used by Carole, expert/information power used in negotiating with and persuading Mrs Jakes that the ideas presented were sound, and should be put to the governors for consideration. Knowledge is power, and the more informed a person is, the greater influence is their bargaining power. So being adequately prepared for the meeting with Mrs Jakes and the governors was crucial. It prevented Carole from being caught off guard and appearing uninformed.

Negotiating skills were also very important. Fisher *et al.* (1992) in their book *Getting to Yes* argue that every person is a negotiator, because negotiation is a fact of life. 'Everyone negotiates something, every day.' Negotiation is the basic means of getting what you want from others. While negotiation takes place every day, it is not easy to do well. Indeed, Dirschel (1996) believes that few nurses are expert negotiators. Success depends on being systematically prepared, staying calm and self-assured (part of the self-assurance comes from, at least partly, being adequately prepared for the negotiation) and utilizing negotiation tactics. Carole and Mr Crow used flattery and seduction in their negotiations by suggesting that Mrs Jakes had a key role to play in the developments, the objective being to divert the attention of the other party and imply future promises. In this instance, Carole and Mr Crow were able to divert Mrs Jakes's attention from the actual detail of practice developments being suggested, focusing on the role she would have, and implying future kudos for the school.

The outcome was very successful – acceptance that the ideas were sound and access to the governors. Carole and Mr Crow won their case and yet were able to make Mrs Jakes feel satisfied with the outcome; they successfully managed to 'get to yes'.

◯ Case study 4: power to the people

After three weeks of meetings with people, listening patiently to their views about the best way forward, Fay was still at a loss to know how best to develop her new role. Although she had worked in occupational health nursing for the past 10 years, this new role, providing health care to farm workers in a rural setting, was very different from anything she had encountered before. Fay remembered how when she had first started working for Fast-Freeze, her working week was clearly mapped out for her. Now six years later, she was expected to decide what to do and how to do it.

To be fair, the Health Action Zone had clearly articulated why it had created the post and what the immediate priorities were, but this role was very different to working in a single factory or industry, where the workforce was a captive audience. Agriculture and the workings of rural communities were not something completely alien to Fay, as her parents owned a nearby farm, on which she and her brother had grown up. She was glad to be back in the countryside of her birth, away from the hustle and bustle of city life. Indeed, this was one of the reasons she applied for the post in the first place.

Fay stared out of the window of her office on the second floor of the local clinic building, which overlooked the town centre market. As she watched the locals going about their business, she started to think about the priorities, and how she might even begin to make a start addressing them. She was acutely aware that agriculture was an industry in turmoil, with food scares, interference from Brussels, rising debts and reduced productivity. In 1999, farmers saw their profits halved, while the amount of paperwork and bureaucracy increased (BBC 1999a). This, in turn, had resulted in rising stress levels amongst farmers and their families, and increasing rates of suicide. In 1999 almost one farmer per week took his own life (BBC 1999b). These growing health concerns were further compounded by the threats to rural life such as rising fuel costs and the increasing centralization of services, including post offices, banks, and even health care facilities.

Fay sat down at her desk and started to map out on a piece of paper the priority areas. She realized that there was a need to provide local health screening for farmers and their families, especially as many of them lived a considerable distance from GP services. She began to scribble about what the problems with this would be, and quickly identified issues around access, identifying those most in need, and the scope and timing of any intervention. The second issue Fay identified was the need for health promotion, and again she identified issues around access and timing. Finally, she identified the need to develop a coherent strategy around accident prevention. This was a problematic area, not only because of access, but because Fay essentially had no jurisdiction over farmers, who were self-employed.

As she looked up at the clock on the wall in front of her desk, she realized it was after 5.00 p.m., so she quickly packed up her papers and left the office. As she drove home, she passed several farmers and noticed that the farm workers were busy harvesting the crops. Clearly, theirs was a not a nine to five job, and Fay realized that to be successful, hers wouldn't be either. She realized that for the past three weeks of her induction, she had spent time meeting local counsellors and other community workers and finding out what they felt the needs of local agricultural workers were. As she pulled into the driveway of her cottage, she realized that her first piece of work had to be to find out what the farmers and farm workers actually wanted from her.

The following day, Fay set about arranging to collect the views of potential service users. In order to achieve this, she set about making contact by letter with all the farms in her area. She invited people to contact her by letter to make their views known, as well as informing people that she would be canvassing their views at the cattle market each Tuesday and Thursday. Fay also spoke to her parents to identify local frameworks that might be useful points for first contact. Her mother and father pointed out that many of the farmers' wives met up at the local Women's Institute on a monthly basis. Fay arranged to contact the area organizer to see if she could make a short presentation about her role. After several weeks of networking, she was able to organize her first focus group, which was held in the upstairs room of the local public house. She managed to get the Health Action Zone manager to fund a buffet and provide light refreshments for the focus group. Nine people attended the first focus group, which proved to be a very lively discussion.

Fay was delighted with the outcome of the first user consultation, as it had helped her to identify several key principles that she could use as a basis for subsequent service development. The key messages that people had put across were the need for a very flexible service, accessible outside of traditional hours and including health checks at home, both at the break of dawn and at the end of the day. Many people saw market days as a major opportunity to meet people who might need help, as well as providing ample opportunity for ad hoc health assessment and health promotion.

Over the next few months, Fay continued to meet with local people and groups to ascertain their views on service provision. At the same time, she worked to establish some of the services already identified, including home health checks offered at flexible times. Fay started to offer these health checks to people who had not seen their family doctor in the last three years. Additionally, she attended each cattle market to offer health checks to farm workers. The sessions were provided from the Health Promotion caravan and they proved popular, because they allowed access to a service at convenient times. Fay also started to offer health checks using the caravan at some of the larger farms, which employed a number of workers.

Primary and community health care services are for the majority of people the first point of contact with the NHS, and more people receive this form of care than any other in the UK. User views are particularly important because of the complex nature of primary and community care. There is a cumulative body of evidence that local people and service users have very different views on health, health services and priorities to those individuals providing the service. Criticism continues to be levelled at health care professionals for setting health agendas without consulting the public in any meaningful way. The Griffiths Report back in 1983 (DHSS 1983) identified how poor the NHS was at obtaining user's views, and it has become an increasingly important phenomenon. Indeed the government's aim is to build a modern and dependable health service, providing a fast and responsive high quality service. The government has identified that 'listening and responding to the needs of those who use the NHS is an important part of making effective change' (Department of Health 1997a).

Identifying user perspectives on health care is one way in which perceptual gaps between patients and professionals can be lessened. It is a method of attempting to match services more closely to user needs, and providing holistic pictures of the complex systems of health care that users experience.

As this case study demonstrates, the overall intention is to provide the trigger for change in promoting appropriate and efficient health care for local people, which reduces inequalities and addresses the issue of access. Fay as a professional had been given a remit to develop a service, and had met with professionals from other agencies to begin this process. However she very quickly realized that the contacts she had made and priorities that she had begun to map out, together with the expected 9 a.m. to 5 p.m. working hours might not be appropriate. She became quickly aware that in order to develop a flexible, responsive and accessible

Table 6.1 The value of greater public participation in the NHS

Benefits to the NHS
- restoration of public confidence;
- improved outcomes for individual patients;
- more appropriate use of health services;
- potential for greater cost effectiveness;
- contribution to problem resolution;
- sharing with the public responsibilities for health.

Benefits to people
- better outcomes of treatment and care;
- an enhanced sense of self-esteem and capacity to control their own lives;
- a more satisfying experience of using health services;
- improved health;
- a greater sense of ownership of the NHS.

Benefits to public health
- reduction in health inequalities;
- improved health;
- greater understanding of the links between health and circumstances in which people live their lives;
- more healthy environmental, social and economic policies.

Benefits to communities and to society as a whole
- improved social cohesion;
- a healthier democracy – reducing the democratic deficit;
- a health service better able to meet the needs of citizens;
- more attention to cross-cutting policy issues and closer cooperation between agencies with a role to play in health improvement.

Both health and health care are improved by participation.

Source: Developed from DoH (1998e)

service, the farmers' views were crucial. One of the most important principles demonstrated in this case study in seeking the views of users, is that their perspective must have credibility and authority at least equal to the perspective of those who manage, run or provide health care.

The value of greater public participation in the NHS is summarized in the document *In the Public Interest: Developing a Strategy for Public Participation in the NHS* (Department of Health 1998e). This is outlined in Table 6.1.

There is a range of methods of engaging with users of health services and obtaining their views. Surveys, public meetings, complaints/suggestions schemes, service-user forums, focus groups, opinion polls, neighbourhood forums, citizen panels or juries are to name but a few (Audit Commission 1999b). Fay concentrated upon establishing some networks with local farmers and their families, making herself available within the environment in which they lived and worked. By doing this, she was able to establish a rapport and some understanding of who she was, and what she was trying to achieve. She was then able to go on and develop focus groups with the farming community on the basis of the relationship she had established.

Focus groups are a particularly effective method of obtaining users' views. Their strength lies in exploring attitudes, perceptions and experiences. Focus groups are, in fact, group interviews, generally involving eight to twelve individuals who discuss a particular topic under the direction of a moderator. In some sense, they are more than a group interview, because they actually rely on interaction with the group. Krueger (1988) argues that the fundamental stance of this method is that attitudes and perceptions relating to products, services or programmes are developed in part by interactions with people. Group interactions produce information and insights that would be less accessible without the interaction found in the group. Group processes can help people explore and clarify their views, examining not only what people think, but how they think and why they think in that way. The main advantage of focus groups is the opportunity to observe and collect a large amount of data in a limited period of time. The combined effort of the group produces a wider range of information, insights and ideas than could be secured from an accumulation of responses from a number of individuals secured privately. Vigilant facilitation is required, so that participants do not talk over one another, and get side-tracked from the topic under discussion. In the field of health, the major advantage of focus groups as a means of obtaining user views is that they do not discriminate against people who cannot read or write, and can encourage participation from people who are reluctant to be interviewed on their own, or who feel they have nothing to say (Kitzinger 1995).

In conclusion, within the NHS we have witnessed a paradigm shift to the empowerment model, where users of health services are no longer passive recipients of care. We have moved beyond the impasse of consumerism, to an environment that promotes genuine user empowerment. Involving users is challenging work for community nurses, but is an extremely powerful tool for designing and improving the quality and effectiveness of services, and in particular ensuring that as service providers we stay in touch with citizens.

◯ Conclusion

The case studies presented in this chapter together reflect the importance and the impact of power and influence on practice development. Collectively, they identify issues that can facilitate the process, in particular those that provide a positive force for change, and also those barriers that present obstacles to development.

Case study 1 focused upon conflict, demonstrating the power of collaboration and the positive influence that working together can bring. This case study identified how collaboration unlocks professionals from conflict that can otherwise stifle and stagnate development. Case study 2 described the shift to a primary care-led NHS and the imbalance in power between nurses and doctors. It highlighted the importance of true partnership working, and the need for cooperation in redressing and overcoming the barriers, established over many years, that can so easily prevent change and development from happening. Case study 3 identified the power of negotiation in an instance where there is a complete imbalance of power in a relationship. Case study 4 described the very powerful impact user perspectives can have on practice development. It identifies the value and importance of engaging with users and obtaining their views in ensuring that when practice is developed it is done in a way that is acceptable and appropriate to users, providing responsive, flexible and accessible services.

There is no doubt that in the current complex, turbulent and often confusing environment in which community nurses work, understanding the impact of power and how to be influential is crucial to leading, implementing and managing the process of practice development.

(7) It ain't what you do, it's the way that you do it: new and different approaches to practice

Kate Henderson-Nichol

◯ Chapter summary

This chapter describes examples of developments in practice in four of the community nursing specialisms. It paints a very compelling and colourful picture of community nurses who seek more effective ways of meeting the needs of their client group. The process that such practitioners go through is vividly described and the issues that they face are explored. Readers are encouraged to read each case study and not concentrate solely on the ones that relate to their own community nursing specialism. The themes that emerge from each, namely networking and communication, evidence, leadership and empowerment, are important and can be translated to any sphere of practice development.

◯ Case study 1: care in custody – myth or manageable?

Police flanked either side of a youth of 19 years old who gazed expressionless into the solemn eyes of the stipendiary magistrate as he pronounced the sentence. The court officials grimly shuffled through the papers, ready for the next sunken-eyed prisoner to slouch into the dock. Andrew's mother broke down in tears, shaking her head in despair. Standing on her own, she was the butt of hatred and verbal abuse from a middle-aged lady whose son had been brutally assaulted with lighted matches, and who was subsequently hospitalized for a considerable length of time. The victim was unlikely to regain the vision in his left eye, and his handsome good looks were gone forever. A frenzied attack, all for a wallet with £25 in it and a watch, that turned out to be a fake anyway. Both women were in tears, one in fury on behalf of her son's loss of life potential, and the other at the loss of her boy. Whatever happened to that happy, football-crazed kid, whose ambition had changed within such a short time from wanting to play for Manchester United, to wanting to fill his body with filth? Her other son, who had been at the receiving end of several batterings as a result of Andrew's habit, was fast approaching the age when Andrew had first experimented (as far as she knew) with a couple of Es. After that, the odd spliff had become a regular activity, then came the late nights, the all-night disappearances. The mood swings had been intolerable. Andrew's schoolwork deteriorated rapidly, until he was expelled and there were constant rows at home which were tearing the family apart. Then the money and ornaments started disappearing. He had wanted for nothing as a young child, so what happened? She blamed herself entirely. If only she had stopped smoking in her early pregnancy, but she hadn't known she was pregnant till 13 weeks gestation. The crowd he had got in with was a far cry from the adolescence she had envisaged for her boy. Perhaps she should have locked him in his room like her husband had wanted. If only she had been a better mother. Tormented for a lifetime ahead, she left the courtroom reflecting on where she thought she had gone wrong, leaving behind her son who was to be locked into a room with no escape.

Alcohol and substance misuse is a scourge of today's society, annihilating many a family's hopes and aspirations. No selector of class or creed, its menacing lure prevails upon the innocent, the vulnerable and the reckless. The consequences of drug activity were summarized by the UK's first anti-drugs coordinator, Keith Hellawell (Home Office 1998b: 38): 'The social, economic, psychological, crime and health-related costs are formidable. The latest Government-funded research suggests that annual costs, arising from the most serious drug misusers alone, are well over £4 billion.'

While the financial implications are important, so are the human implications. The emotional and physical devastation drugs and alcohol-related crime brings upon families and communities is boundless. Alcohol is a factor in 50 per cent of all crime. Although the influence of alcohol tends to be overshadowed by drug-related issues, the consequences are equally as far-reaching. Gossop *et al.* (1998) state that the National Treatment Outcome Research Study (NTORS) is the largest and most robust study of drug treatment services in the UK. It reported that following treatment, the use of opiates more than halved and there was a considerable decrease in use of quantity and frequency with those still using drugs. The two key findings relating to this project were that overall, psychological and physical health improved and there was a reduction in criminal behaviour. The estimate offered by NTORS is that for every

£1 spent on treatment, £3 could be saved within the criminal justice system alone.

However, the stark reality is that gangs of youths, mostly males, huddle together on street corners, down alleys, or tucked away in car parks and municipal parks, where they fill their bodies with toxins in the name of 'having nothing better to do' or 'having a laugh'. Alcohol, drugs and youth make a dangerous cocktail. The precipitator of daring acts of 'bravery', such as mugging an elderly person on his way back home from bingo just for the princely sum of £5, or perhaps setting light to an empty warehouse for the pleasure of destruction, are typical examples of a rise in alcohol and drug-related crime. It is not unusual wherever one walks in towns at night to see young people, male and female, sprawled drunk against walls clutching half-empty brandy bottles and beer cans. Lolling from side to side, they avoid their vomit in the road, and laugh hysterically as they enjoy their freedom within their gangs, while they plan their next moves that will undoubtedly pave their route to the police station.

In 1998 a Home Office study (Edmonds *et al.* 1998) found that 61 per cent of arrestees tested positively for at least one illegal drug. This figure was applied to a needs analysis undertaken in Lancaster and Morecambe with their arrest data for 1997 demonstrating an expectation of up to eight arrestees per day in this area. The snapshot of evidence in their district over a weekend period of their 55 arrests, showed 72 per cent were under the influence of drugs and/or alcohol.

But how can health care services access these people? They are notoriously difficult to reach, as they are often outside formal education systems and are invariably without employment. Many are well known to the criminal justice system and probation services, with many being frequenters of HM prison services, where it is estimated that two-thirds of prisoners have severe alcohol problems. Many of these people are eventually referred to specialist services, when their drug and/or alcohol habit is firmly entrenched in their way of life, making the benefits of preventive work virtually impossible, and leaving damage limitation the only viable option. It makes sense to try and help this group of people access specialist services as early as possible to help them live drug-free lives. Surely a planned, proactive approach would be an answer?

The case study highlights how Andrew would have been an ideal candidate for a proactive custody-based service, had there been one operational at the time. He, like many before him, sat in his cell shuddering in cold turkey, terrified at the prospect of his impending court appearance, where he was about to receive his first custodial sentence, and where he knew his mother would be weeping in desperation and disappointment. His father had refused to attend court, but perhaps that was because he had trashed his parents' suburban home and broken his brother's nose in the rage to find the extra money just for that last line to sniff. He was in the system now, and it is detainees like him who need support and encouragement to change destructive health-related behaviour. Avril, previously a community psychiatric nurse in the alcohol team at the Bay Community NHS Trust in Lancashire, recognized this need and set out to find a way to address it.

Being in custody is traumatic, and it is also a time when being confined in a small place and looking at the cell walls provides inescapable time. This can be an opportunity for arrestees to reflect on the consequences of their actions. It is a critical window of opportunity for health services and police to work together, just at the time when the client's motivation to change might be higher than when they're on the outside. It is a window of opportunity to be grasped and entered. Avril discussed with her colleagues the idea of accessing clients who were in custody as a result of allegedly undertaking alcohol-related crimes by paging community psychiatric nurses in the Community Alcohol Team. Discussing it at length with her police colleagues at sergeant level, she was met with enthusiasm and commitment to take a service forward. The painful fact was, that for all the dedication to improve services, it never took off because there was no 'power-house' behind the scheme. The obstacle was that the levels of sister and sergeant were not senior enough to negotiate, plan and implement a collaborative service development. But Avril never gave up believing that nurses could make a difference for this client group.

Within three months of her promotion to Substance Misuse Manager, the annual round of bids for the Lancashire Joint Finance Initiative between the health authority and local authority were invited. Now a manager, Avril was keen to further develop a substantive working relationship with the police. Not backwards in coming forwards, she had already been making headway with her police colleagues at Detective Chief Inspector (DCI) level, through the Drug Reference Group and the Community Safety and Drugs Working Group, which is a subgroup of the Crime and Disorder Strategy Group. She wanted to access clients earlier – the sooner the better. That meant improving communication and collaborative working practices with the courts, probation and prison services, as well as with the police, at operational and strategic levels.

Evidence suggests that arrest referral schemes seeking to put users in touch with treatment agencies improve access to services. However Avril wanted to progress this further by taking treatment into the custody suites; as Newburn and Elliott (1998) suggest, arrest referral schemes are more successful when the drug worker is placed within the custody suite, rather than relying on the police to page for services.

Based on this and other supporting evidence, Avril and her team decided to bid for joint finance to develop this collaborative service. She continued liaising with senior police officers at DCI level, who in turn canvassed their most senior officers in their organization, and subsequently provided local figures to substantiate Avril's proposal to the health authority. Meanwhile, Avril was canvassing the Consultant in Public Health, to whom she presented her evidence on a one-to-one basis, as well as the Trust Manager of Mental Health Services and the Director of Corporate Development. The Bay Community NHS Trust duly submitted the application, along with a separate proposal, containing supporting letters from the police, probation services and the chair of the Drugs Reference Group (DRG). The scheme had already been approved as a priority by the DRG and the consortium was soon successful in its bid for joint finance.

Funding from the Lancashire Joint Finance initiative was allocated for the establishment of a trailblazing service, based within the existing Lancaster and Morecambe Community Drug Team (CDT) and managed by Avril in her capacity as Substance Misuse Manager, in conjunction with a multiagency steering group. As this is a three-year project, there is a substantive evaluation process in place, which will be essential to securing further funding to ensure a long-term future for this provision. The Crime Foundation, a consultancy employed by the Lancashire Constabulary, is evaluating the impact upon crime and community safety, while two independent researchers, Nick Bowles and Robert Monks, are undertaking responsibility for the evaluation of health gain, service user perspectives and interagency working. Three registered nurses are now employed in the project, two are based within Lancaster and Morecambe police stations, while the third provides the interface between the CDT and the courts, probation and the prison services. In addition, the three nurses operate an on-call system that ensures weekend cover for each police station.

The first of its kind in the UK, this service offers a full nursing assessment to all arrestees to ascertain their physical, psychological and psychological status. This is what makes it different from straightforward arrest referral schemes. It has been a source of frustration for Avril and her colleagues that people have assumed the service is arrest referral. Although there are overlaps between the two concepts, arrest referral schemes tend to use non-clinical staff who encourage arrestees to take up services, but they may then end up in a queue. This custody intervention service takes treatment to the cells in the custody suite, which means that arrestees receive a full nursing assessment of their mental and physical health, which addresses issues of dual diagnosis (mental health and substance misuse problems). The nurses have therefore become an important resource for the police. This availability of nursing care for detainees has resulted in custody officers commenting positively that they are now able to link detainees to a nursing service immediately, which means that they, as officers of the law, can provide more than just a processing system for their arrestees. The nurse, who is based in the custody suite, engages the user into a treatment programme. That same nurse becomes the 'named nurse' throughout the programme, as she/he coordinates and delivers care and provides all the liaison services required at subsequent stages of involvement with the criminal justice system, thus establishing a health pathway for the detainees.

Avril and her colleagues are well aware that not every arrestee will accept the offer of treatment programmes, but for a group who are virtually impossible to access in the first place, as a 'captive' audience in custody, detainees can at least have a choice. The service is offered to all arrestees, and those who decline to engage with treatment are provided with health promotion information with a view to limitation of harm.

Networking and communication skills have been the critical success factors in Avril's negotiations between two very different organizations, and it has taken time and patience to persuade her colleagues in health that it is 'safe' to consult and share information with the police without breaking confidentiality. There have been a lot of traditional barriers to challenge, especially around the issue of confidentiality, but gradually, as time has passed and myths about each profession dispelled, the team works together collaboratively. Support for nurses working within a police environment has raised issues for their management, but regular clinical supervision from their team leader has proved to be invaluable in assisting each nurse to feel totally part of the Drugs and Alcohol Team.

This custody intervention service provides care for one of the most difficult client groups to access. It took visionary leadership and exemplary communication skills to make it work. Initial findings suggest that it is a scheme that could be disseminated and implemented UK-wide, especially in the light of the current policy emphasis on men's health and prison health care.

◯ Case study 2: dying to stay at home

Sandy's role as district nurse supporting Marie, who was principal carer for her ailing and elderly mother, was becoming blurred with the memories of her own experience of nursing a chronically sick parent. Although several years had elapsed, Sandy would always carry the burden of guilt as she recalled the rasping struggle her mother had in the fight for breath against emphysema. Failed promises echoed in her ears, that no parent of hers would ever need to be cared for, or die, in a hospital or a nursing home. But the sad reality was, that for Sandy's mother, the promise was broken. Tears welled up in her eyes as she remembered that day her mother was taken to hospital. The clash of the ambulance doors still rang in her ears, combated by the cruel sense of relief that the burden of care was at last to be shared. Her torment was that it was neither her mother's wish nor Sandy's that she would ever leave her home and familiar surroundings. Two hours postadmission, Sandy's mother was dead.

Seeing Marie caring for her mother, Elizabeth, was the mirror image of her own situation. Elizabeth had suffered from multiple sclerosis for 12 years and was now completely bedridden – and determined to remain at home. Sandy and Marie had talked long and hard and although Marie was greatly appreciative of all the support Sandy and her colleagues could offer, it didn't alleviate the burden of care that invariably rests with relatives. Marie's career had been about to take off. The senior partner of the legal firm where she was a successful legal secretary had offered her the opportunity, with full funding, to undertake training to become a legal executive. Her career prospects were exceptionally good but, under the circumstances, she opted to give up her job to care for her mother. She was torn between trying to 'do the right thing' and care for her mother at home, while constantly battling with her feelings of resentment at the sacrifice she had made. The notion of nursing homes was a painful one for her, especially as her mother was so desperately opposed to it, but she knew that as things were at present, she simply could not cope.

It seemed so unfair that for Elizabeth there was nothing in the way of special care at home – just like for Sandy's mum there had been nowhere for her to be cared for, other than an acute hospital. Marie knew someone two streets away who was dying from cancer, and her family, who were the main carers, were receiving Hospice at Home services, as well as the Marie Curie nursing service. While sorry to hear about this family, Marie felt in a way that they were the 'lucky' ones. She often asked why people identify with the pain of cancer more than the interminable suffering from other conditions like MS and emphysema? Sandy could offer no answer, but it preyed on her mind.

Sandy spent a considerable amount of time wrestling with social services to increase their support for Marie and Elizabeth, but to no avail. Her colleagues at the health centre agreed that it was time to step up the amount of visits from three to four per day, in an attempt to provide more support. But Sandy really did understand what Marie was experiencing, and knew that this was tokenism and would not address the main issues. Sandy returned to Elizabeth to tell her that the visits would be increased day and night.

Typical of a day in district nursing, Sandy left Marie and Elizabeth, who were her last clients, at 5.15 p.m., called into a supermarket for a sandwich, and headed straight for the Primary Care Group (PCG) meeting.

Unable to get her last clients out of her mind as she waited in a traffic jam at roadworks, she suddenly wondered what the point was of attending a meeting that would be focusing on overgenerous staffing levels in her health centre. The roadworks cleared, but her head did not. She could not rationalize the lack of support for her patients and she clearly had not resolved her own experience. As the meeting progressed, her attention was suddenly drawn to Mark Sanderson, one of the commissioning managers from the health authority, who outlined the priorities for the Elderly Health Improvement Programme (HImP). He invited the group to consider proposals designed to prevent unnecessary hospital and nursing home admissions. Now this was her chance to influence change.

The meeting had come to an abrupt end, but the gauntlet was down. Sandy caught up with Mark Sanderson and described the experiences that she and her colleagues had on a day-to-day basis of caring for families who were nursing chronically and terminally sick relatives. She was articulate and precise, knowing exactly how to emphasize the benefits for patients, carers and the NHS in providing the quality and level of support to keep patients out of hospital. Presented with such a rational argument, Mark advised that Sandy should liaise with Diane, the PCG Service Development Manager, to discuss the possibility of putting together a bid for funding for a project to address the issue of support for caring for patients at home who have diagnoses other than cancer.

Sandy's proposal clearly had an impact on the commissioning manager, for when she contacted Diane, the Service Development Manager, she had already been briefed and was drafting some ideas ready for Sandy when she rang. As she put the appointment in her diary for the meeting, Sandy was overcome with a feeling that, perhaps in the future, she could be absolved from the guilt she carried for her mum's admission into hospital. It felt like a journey towards her own atonement.

Here was the opportunity for her to be a real advocate for the hundreds of other families like hers that were suffering in the same way. Covering Sandy's work for the afternoon that she met with Diane was difficult, but the possibility of being able to change and develop practice meant that everyone was starting to pull together with a common objective. The need for a Hospice at Home service was clearly identifiable and implicit in practice, but there was no empirical evidence on which to base a service. Diane wanted to know the numbers involved, so Sandy's first task was to undertake a mapping exercise. With her colleagues' assistance, she undertook a telephone survey of practitioners to ask how many of their patients would benefit from such a service. A picture emerged of an evidence base, and included in that evidence base was of course Marie and her mother. Sandy had not said anything to Marie about the level of progress in the impending proposals, other than to discuss her views about such a service. Marie had responded, as expected, to her questions, and although the increased level of visits was appreciated, it was not the same type of support as could be provided by hospice care at home. However Marie felt that at last someone was listening to her, and perhaps in the not too distant future she too would benefit from such a service, and be able to pick up her career again.

Sandy and Diane pored over the data presented and examined the types of non-cancer conditions that required community services, the type of support provided and the impact of the situation and level of support on carers. Sandy found that she was using Marie in particular as a case study, vividly explaining how it really is for patients and their carers. In Elizabeth and Marie's case, it had always been their expressed wish that a nursing home was out of the question, but in the circumstances they found themselves, there was no choice. The empathy forged between Sandy, Diane and Marie (whose identity was kept confidential during all discussions) was tangible, as the practitioner and manager worked together to create plans for a better system of care. They were searching to design a service that would offer families the choice to be nursed at home, equal to that offered for patients suffering from cancer.

As Sandy and Diane began to put together a proposal, they were interrupted by Sandy's mobile telephone. It was Marie. Her mother had just died. The meeting was curtailed and Sandy went straight to Marie's house. This was certainly food for thought for the manager, reminding her of her own practical experience as a district nurse, now buried in the mists of time. While Sandy went to her patient's aid, Diane started to plan strategically about how and when they should present the proposal to the PCG/health authority meeting.

Six weeks went by before they could present their bid, which Diane led. Diane had warned Sandy that others might not be as enthusiastic as they were about the plans, and, sure enough, the main hostility came from a local chest physician – particularly during Diane's formal presentation. There were interesting dynamics in that meeting. The power of the hostility began to drive the mood amongst the audience. The physician was firm and articulate, and contested the need for such a service, on the grounds that existing services provided in local hospitals were of high quality and that their complaint record was negligible. The strength of feeling lurched to his side and Sandy sensed that she and Diane were losing ground fast. She passed a note to Diane, asking that she be given the chance to address the meeting, to give a practitioner's view. Diane stopped the debate about existing service provision and invited Sandy to state her case. Sandy stood before the meeting and began with,

> How would you feel if your mum begged you not to 'put her in a home because she'd die?' The problem is that your mum, who has

cared for you all your life, always put you first, was there uncondi-
tionally through your good and bad times, has protected you from
harm, has cared for you when you were ill and would lay down
her life for you . . . and she is now ill, incontinent, immobile and
depressed. She begs you to help her and, above all, not send her
away. She wants to be at home, where her family life has always
been. How do you feel? What would you do?

The assembled group went quiet and waited for the answer. Suddenly, the reality of what was being proposed came to life. The silent
reflection was obvious, as people thought about their own parents and
tried to imagine them with that kind of dependency. Sandy continued
her graphic depiction of a real-life situation. She told the story of the
struggle Marie had with her mother, Elizabeth, through the last years of
her deteriorating life, until her recent uncomfortable death. But her
death saved her from what she perceived as the worst experience of all,
in fading away in a nursing home, away from her precious family and
memories. She had had enough to come to terms with in having a
disabling condition that rendered her bedfast and incontinent, without
the added indignity of living in a place not of her own choice. She
always said that, even though her body had given up its ghost, there
was nothing at all wrong with her mental capacity and she lived the life
of a prisoner within a ruin. Elizabeth had been powerless and the service provision was about to wield its own power and control over the
vulnerable.

As Sandy spoke with the eloquence of the Bar, the mood of the
meeting changed, as they began to imagine what it would have been
like for Elizabeth, or their own parent, to end up in long-term care –
surely an ill-informed decision, resulting in a negative outcome. She
finished with, 'I ask you to consider, could you sleep at night – or would
you want something different for your family?'

Sandy sat down, with the aplomb of a defence barrister, to a tangible
silence. As the audience thought about what they had heard, a more
positive mood emerged. The physician launched another attack, but was
put firmly back in his place by the rest of the group. The outcome was
positive, in that the health authority agreed to consider the possibility
for funding, and they would let Diane know in due course.

Three weeks later Diane was informed that the proposal had been
accepted. The next strategic move came in the form of an advertisement
for a coordinator for the new service, which was to be piloted over two
years, and have an integral evaluation strategy through links with the
local university. Sandy applied and was successful. Based in a health
centre, she established the service to include support workers who
were to provide assistance with washing, dressing and sitting services,

including night shifts. A training programme was developed and implemented for support workers on basic nursing skills, for example moving
and handling, hand washing, disease processes and treatment, skin care
and wound care management. The district nurses involved in managing
care worked as a team and developed an evaluation tool to obtain user
perspectives. A researcher from the university was collating the data and
creating a portfolio of evidence.

Six months into the project, the social services Home Care Manager
decided to remove all home carers on the grounds that the in-year
budget was such that cuts had to be made. The philosophy was that
rather than reduce provision, their removal of home carers simply shifted
the responsibility for care from social to health services. There had been
no negotiation for this move, and the once shared objectives seemed to
have disappeared, along with the home carers. Not to be defeated, Sandy
met with the Community Care Manager, and using her negotiating
skills, entered into a series of discussions over a period of five months.
Having presented some initial findings compiled by the researcher, she
persuaded the manager that, rather than reducing service provision,
they should be working together, and the discussions revolved around
resetting joint objectives. These were based on examination of the patients' needs and of the skills of the support workers and home carers,
which were to become pooled and shared to reduce overlap, but their
specialist skills were to be respected and utilized to their full potential.

The outcome has been that a greater flexibility of service provision
is available for patients with chronic non-cancer conditions than are
offered outside the traditional models of care. The cost effectiveness has
been proven in terms of a huge reduction in overlap, between home
carers and hospice workers, as the latter will make meals and undertake
other duties while in the patient's home.

It took a deep understanding of patients' and carers' needs and exemplary communication skills to initiate this project. Sandy and her team
succeeded, with the result that patients and carers in her PCG have the
dignity of choice of a tailor-made service.

This case study highlights several issues. First, the notion of experience
as a valuable source of evidence for possible development is highlighted.
This was discussed earlier in Chapter 2. Essentially, experience is used
by Sandy to both identify the need for the development, and to support
the selling of the idea to the HImP group. Second, the study clearly
illustrates how a change agent may influence a group. In the case study,
Sandy and Diane experience difficulties in presenting their case for change
to the HImP group, because of the influence of the consultant physician.
Without doubt, the influence exerted by the physician within the group
is likely to be related to power. Power, as both a factor in influencing

and stifling development, is discussed in detail by Wendy Burke in Chapter 6. Despite the negative influence that the physician was able to exert over the group, Sandy and Diane were ultimately successful in achieving funding for the development. Group conformity is an important issue in practice development, as this can make or break any development. Conformity amongst group members has been well documented (King and Anderson 1995). However, most of the studies to date have demonstrated that groups exert pressures to conform with a majority position. King and Anderson (1995: 69) describe how conformity can be seen to result from two interrelated factors:

- informational – we look to others to explain things to us;
- normative – we look to others for an indication of what is expected of us.

While there has been a wealth of social psychology research examining conformity as a result of majority influence, there has been less attention paid to how one or two individuals can influence the decisions of a group. Studies by Moscovici (1976) identified how minorities could succeed in changing the position of the majority. King and Anderson (1995: 70) suggest a minority can influence the majority in a group if they

- present a consistent and coherent argument;
- present a view that is consistent with the insider viewpoint.

The case study suggests that Sandy was able to use her experience as both a district nurse and from caring for her mother to present an insider's viewpoint. By getting members of the group to think of how they might feel in a similar situation, Sandy was able to convince the group that her proposal was consistent with the aims of the health improvement programme and therefore a development worthy of funding.

◯ Case study 3: a tide of change

Dogged by poverty, crime, alcohol and substance abuse, division between two grim estates in this tourist haven on the south coast further compounded social isolation. It was the last place on earth where people wanted to be housed. If you got a place there, you really had hit rock bottom. It was the same for the health visitors. You knew you were put there because no one else wanted to be, and you were usually covering long-term sickness. The average burn-out rate was two years, with replacement by inexperienced health visitors, who further compounded the statistics of stress related illness, and so the situation droned on – for all parties.

The residents viewed the health visitors with contempt, to say the least. These interfering busybodies were regarded as coming from the 'social', and policing their childcare, their families and their lives. In addition to health visiting, other services offered typically included housing officers, social workers, Community Education Workers and various voluntary agencies such as Women's Aid and Samaritans. They all had a part to play, but with dubious effectiveness because they invariably overlapped in their contacts with the families, lulling them into a fantasy that they were providing coordinated services. A medley of services does not equate with planned, coordinated and effective care. In fact, they were all working in isolation with their own agendas and providing the service as described in their job descriptions. Their focus was therefore on process and not outcomes.

The picture is one of divisiveness and desperation. In the early 1990s, a mini-riot in the area sparked off a whole series of negative media coverage. Not surprisingly, the residents rose to their community's defence and decided that it was time the outside world changed its perception of their estate, and they issued a challenge to the negative assumptions in a bid to stop the continuous victimization. There was no doubt that the estate bore all the dubious qualities the media loves to revel in. It boasted a ghetto environment of high violent and petty crime figures, appalling poverty and deprivation, high truancy rates, early teenage pregnancy and a raft of poverty-related disease and ill-health statistics. The streets were not safe by day or night; violence was rife.

The negative media coverage turned out to be the catalyst for change, however. In response to the press stories, a core of disgruntled residents decided that it was time the outside world changed its perception of the estate as a 'dysfunctional' community. They invited both statutory and voluntary agencies to help in their quest to relabel the estate and help make the community something people wanted to become part of.

Despite the negative environment for health visiting practice, there was no lack of will on their part in wishing things were better. A far cry from the public health emphasis of their training, the reality was that health visitors experienced a widening theory–practice gap that was swallowing them up in a catch-up culture of wading through endless lists of overdue tasks. Rapid staff turnover invariably meant that the new blood would have its ardour quelled in time to adopt the 'keeping things ticking over' mentality of practice. The result was a wealth of stifled and wasted skills, accompanied by the inevitable demotivation. Despite this, there was still sense among the health visitors that they really wanted to contribute to and help this community. There was also an inevitable frustration that 'they' (the health visitors) were not accepted. Typically, organizational barriers and the paralysing 'professional versus patient' concept had caused an impasse, only to be challenged by the mini-riot on the estate, which precipitated a catalogue of change as its residents stood up and demanded to be heard.

For sustainable change to occur, it needs to be managed by skilled leadership, which will promote adoption of the process by all parties working together as a team (West 1999). This project, like any successful community development work, was not about *imposing* significant change onto a community based on assumptions about its needs. The health needs of that stigmatized population had been identified some time before the riot, based on the *Health of the Nation* targets (Department of Health 1992), and the health problems of the community were therefore regarded by professionals as largely self-imposed through lifestyle. There was a culture of it being 'their own fault'.

After residents invited the statutory and voluntary agencies to help them, a survey of the estate was facilitated as part of the health authority's supportive response. It was completed by the residents and related directly to their needs and wishes. The results demonstrated clearly that residents wanted somewhere specific, where there was someone with whom they could identify, to ask for health information and advice. Crucially, in terms of developing community practice, this population saw their health needs as something very different from the 'professional' view, namely as housing, environmental and social issues, rather than disease related conditions.

The residents were not going to let the matter drop and something had to be done. The health authority finally advised the establishment of a post, in which the post holder would look at the survey results and 'do something with that community'. An outsider from the area was appointed as a Community Development Worker (Anna) who had a proven record of successful leadership. She also offered the post a substantial health visiting background and she was committed to public health.

The community development initiated by Anna's appointment was about working in partnership with the residents to create social capital and a healthy community. Facilitating such change required that she first had to get to know the community. As Campbell *et al.* (1999: 4) suggest, promoting 'health-enabling' communities requires an in-depth understanding,

> of the types of community networks, resources and relationships that exist in their local communities of interest, and that their understandings of community resonate with the experiences and perceptions of ordinary people at the grass-roots level.

Focusing on the client group without any hierarchical bias, Anna began talking to people straightaway. She included in her discussions: the residents, health service colleagues, education workers, social workers and housing officers. Relying on her communication skills to influence and negotiate, she employed those essential tools to effect the process of change. Her core specialist and practical experience under-pinned her knowledge that effective communication skills significantly improve health outcomes and also impacted positively on health professionals themselves, in terms of satisfaction with work (Silverman *et al.* 1998). She soon began to engage the community and colleagues alike to reflect on their lives and their practice. Anna began to draw the two together, and saw prejudices dispelled on both sides. The more she facilitated discussion amongst her health visiting and social service colleagues, the more she was able to feed into the conversation, and dir-ectly involve the view of the community with which they were charged to work.

Accessing the community to ascertain its view as a stranger was brave – some would say naïve. You have to have self-belief, stamina and determination to do that. Anna used the survey as the bedrock of her investigations to find out who people were and what they wanted and needed from service providers. Interviews were held in residents' homes, rent offices, playgroups and residents' association meetings, to find out what was important to them and what it was like to live in this particu-lar area. The initial stages of establishing and translating this community development programme into practice thus far required some essential ingredients, transferable to developing any other seedling initiative. To start with, she and her fledgling team had to have a clear purpose, which was becoming obvious from the content of the discussions with the residents. This allegedly dysfunctional community was at an impasse. They wanted things to improve, but exactly what and how took the strength of a leader, and that leader was Anna.

Underpinned by the legitimacy from management her vision clari-fied, and the picture she created in her mind was of a cohesive, self-supporting community, with shared responsibility for health and social care with the residents. She was putting into practice a theory of com-munity development without realizing it. Facilitating a population to work in partnership with statutory and voluntary agencies creates the foundation for the growth of 'social capital', a term that refers to the 'community cohesion that results when a community is characterised by a rich associational life – a variable array of strong social networks' (Campbell *et al.* 1999: 7). The process of managed change developed from the evidence collected in the survey, and from Anna's conversations with residents, health and social care colleagues led to the identification of three core principles:

- leadership;
- listening;
- risk-taking.

It is important to recognize where the term 'managed' fits into the change management process, and not confuse managing with leading. There are similarities between management and leadership, and many people in those positions share skills from each category – but they are inherently different. Zaleznik (1992: 126) states that 'leadership inevitably requires using power to influence the thoughts and actions of other people'.

Anna gradually influenced a culture of 'letting go' of traditional health visiting practice in favour of a community development approach. Her ability to provide a safe environment at a time of perceived professional chaos and disorganization was the key to breaking down the professional barriers that so often paralyse practice development. Slowly and carefully, she helped the wheels of change trundle into action. To lead changing practice Drucker (1996: xii) suggests that the effective leader will ask, 'What needs to be done?' moving on to 'What can and should I do to make a difference?'

Anna continually checked with herself and her new team what their aims and objectives were, what was making it happen and what was blocking progress. Although this became an integrated working partnership with professionals and residents working side by side, it was Anna's vision and drive that motivated and stimulated change. There is often a price to pay for this kind of leadership because feathers are inevitably ruffled, often amongst managers and colleagues alike. It is essential to keep focused and do the right thing for the community. Bennis (1990: 18) in his search for common traits on successful leaders, found that 'Leaders are people who do the right thing; managers are people who do things right'.

Anna's team created an open environment, gnawing away at barriers and establishing trust. Once the process of change was facilitated with a committed team, it developed of its own accord. Over a period of two years, with agencies and residents talking together, a local housing association offered its support with some premises rent-free for a year so the community could access the services they needed. This community flat is now jointly managed by the residents and local agencies. It is in walking distance for all residents, as it is situated on the estate. Residents are offered baby clinics, well persons' clinics, volunteer courses, drop-in advice sessions, housing surgeries, Street Samaritans, Playlink and a variety of family living courses, including cooking on a budget, managing a budget, writing letters, basic computing skills, maths and English.

Anna kept the momentum up, working with health visiting colleagues and identifying the critical success factors of this wider public health role. Local health visitors were never told to work in this way; they adopted it of their own accord as they became integrated into the community. A team spirit was essential for the project's success, which meant everyone taking part in the process from the start. Anna adhered to the principles of creating successful teamwork as described by West (1999: 11) who suggests three key points to consider for teams to work effectively:

1 developing reflexivity (analyse their activity);
2 clear objectives, high levels of communication and participation, and support for innovation;
3 removal of organizational barriers, replaced by support networks.

It was the birth of community spirit, starting from scratch.

As the community developed, wider health issues that needed addressing were raised by residents – such as teenage pregnancy, drug abuse and the sale of cigarettes by ice cream vendors to children. Anna managed to negotiate funding for a community sexual health worker who, while offering access to specialist advice, worked in close liaison with all the other agencies to tackle the problem of teen pregnancy across the broad spectrum of its causes and effects. The battle against drugs and substance misuse is being addressed through the community itself, working with community mental health and social workers and the police.

These residents are no longer regarded as being at the bottom of the heap. *They* are driving their health and social care forward in partnership with statutory and voluntary agencies. The agencies have facilitated change, while the community has developed itself. There is a waiting list to get housed there now – a far cry from the days when it was seen as the last stop before Hell. Anna, who initiated the change process, says there are four crucial points that influenced the change to community development: 'It's about

- not being 'precious' about professional boundaries and specific expertise;
- not being afraid to admit that things have gone wrong, then going back to the drawing board together and all looking at things differently;
- having the ability to share knowledge and communicate around all community work;
- listening to the community, involving them in all stages and working *with* them.

This development was initially motivated by one person who created an environment of change that made people stand back, take stock of their work and reflect on their practice. It is not easy being an innovator and it can be a lonely job to have. Anna discovered that it was essential to learn how to play the political game successfully to ensure change was effected at all levels. Another valuable lesson learned was the necessity of having a comprehensive support network in place for herself, beginning with mentorship throughout the scheme as it developed and practice changed. How did it all happen? Because *all* parties started talking and by working together, the whole community of residents, including the 'professionals', has developed and will continue to do so.

○ Case study 4: mine's a taboo

Michael was a newly appointed learning disability nurse and had argued vehemently for clinical supervision – an innovation in his trust. Now established as a regular monthly session, he had a burning issue to discuss regarding one of his clients with whom he felt he had made a significant breakthrough. Roger was a trained and experienced supervisor, ready to challenge and support his supervisees to reflect on their practice and ensure its quality and appropriateness.

Michael could barely contain himself in his haste to tell his story about Alan, a spectacularly handsome young man with a moderate learning disability who lived in one of the local group homes. Michael had explained that one would struggle to appreciate that Alan had any learning disability at all, with his looks and ability to take himself into town, walk around etc. Unfortunately, these walks had led him to encounter the police, as he had been regularly seeking sex with other men in nearby toilets. He was duly reported to the home staff, and Michael was asked by his manager to stop this behaviour – an objective that Michael was keen and confident to address.

Roger sat listening intently to the story, carefully planning the timing and content of his response. Michael described his concern for Alan, who was a man wanting sexual contact, in this case with other men. Alan was unlikely to meet other men with whom he could engage in sexual contact at his home, and Michael's assessment was that Alan was expressing a legitimate sexual health need and was unaware of the considerable risks he was taking. Michael's clinical experience up to now had revealed that clients' sexuality issues were far from isolated – whatever their preference – and were regarded as rather a tiresome extra that, if ignored or diverted, would in time burn out.

Michael and Alan had met a few times to talk about options and the potential dangers from meeting strangers, particularly under those circumstances. They agreed that the safest solution was for Michael to accompany Alan to a local gay pub. Michael rejoiced in his success, because Alan had really enjoyed himself. Everyone had liked him and he had made a few contacts.

Then came the considered response from Roger, who quietly asked, 'You seem to be pleased with this outcome?' Michael was taken aback for a second and retorted that he was well pleased with such a good result. He was irritated at what he perceived was Roger's lack of comprehension of the magnitude of his intervention, and explained that, by taking Alan to a gay pub, he had ensured that Alan would make homosexual contacts *and* be in a place where he would be sexually valued. Michael was astonished that Roger apparently did not share Michael's enthusiasm for his success. After all, here was a client who had been engaging in an illegal sexual activity – separate from the local gay community – that was disrespectful to him as a person, and who was now empowered to express his sexual needs.

Roger proceeded to explore some of the other risks Michael had discussed with Alan. He was thinking particularly of information on condoms, safe and safer sex. Michael thought this a patronizing question, and retorted that of course Alan wore a condom. But the question came back, 'And is Alan empowered and knowledgeable enough to require that his *partner* wears a condom?'

Michael was suddenly on the spot and beginning to feel uncomfortable. This was not going according to plan, and he replied that he didn't know if Alan would ask his partner to wear protection. Without hesitation, Roger asked what Alan would do if Michael himself approached Alan with offers of sexual favours – would he accept? Michael was incensed at this distorted suggestion, and was uncertain what Roger was driving at. Roger clarified the question and assured him he was asking purely about *Alan's response*, and not commenting on Michael.

Michael thought about it and felt that, hypothetically, it was likely that Alan would be interested. Clearly, as Alan knows Michael is his nurse, Roger suggested that discriminatory skills were an essential component of this scenario. The fact is, Roger explained, that Michael had put Alan, a stunningly good looking young man, in a gay bar, but had not furnished him with the skills to discriminate and make choices on the appropriateness or inappropriateness of sexual partners. Saying 'no' is an acquired skill for people without a learning disability, so how can Alan with a moderate learning disability be expected to do so?

Michael was sinking into his chair, reflecting on his intervention, which he had thought was such a coup for social integration and equality. Clearly he had not thought of the wider implications. He listened to Roger, who quietly suggested that Michael had described to him a young man who indiscriminately had sex with other men. Michael had then colluded with that and put him in a place that he, as his nurse, assumed was better. The problem was that he had increased neither Alan's skills nor ability. His dignity and empowerment remained just the same as when engaging in oral sex in public toilets.

By now Michael was starting to have visions of legal actions against him and media coverage that would paralyse his career. On the other hand, his defence was that he had a valid case, in that Alan, like all clients, was entitled to a full sexual life, whatever their preference, and it would inevitably be a journey where mistakes are made – mistakes not being confined to those with learning disabilities. His mind was leaping by now, when Roger asked about Michael's perception of his 'duty of care to Alan'. Michael spouted the Code of Professional Conduct – which received short shrift. Roger wanted more interpretation than a citation of regulations, at which point Michael suggested that his duty lay in providing Alan with the greatest number of opportunities that will enable him to live as fully as possible, and as independently as possible. Roger questioned whether Michael had in fact done that by taking him to a gay bar. To Michael, the obvious solution had been to extract Alan from illegal sex into safety, where he could meet gay people within his community. Roger asked if Michael really thought that every single one of those members would value and treat Alan appropriately.

Michael conceded that perhaps not *everyone* would treat Alan properly, and he might become the butt of some jokes. Roger was quick to intervene, 'But you said you have met your duty of care?'

By this time Michael's head was spinning. 'Yes!' he had cried. 'I can't *believe* you think it is right to have left him in the toilets – or taken him back to his home where he would have no sex life at all. You really are pissing me off with this. I think I have done something very positive for him – and you are just giving me a load of grief. That somehow, he is this sweet, good looking boy that we must protect from everything. Good care can mean taking good risks.'

Now Roger was getting somewhere with Michael and asked if he really felt it had been a *good* risk. Michael virtually spat that it was, and anyway, what other options were there?

It was at this point that Roger summarized the facts, highlighting three specific problems:

1 Alan is not allowed to have sex at his place of residence.
2 He is not receiving any support for his sexual needs from his home manager or other care staff.
3 Alan was engaged in an illegal sexual activity – possibly not knowing it was illegal or what that implied.

Michael groaned, conceding that perhaps he had not actually analysed each problem. On the other hand, Roger confirmed, the very positive action that Michael had taken was that he had valued Alan's sexual identity – in this case, as a homosexual – and placed him in contact with a community that would also value this, and where he could potentially further develop his sexual experience. Reflecting the question back to Michael again, Roger asked how he viewed the options now.

Michael was calmer and beginning to think much less defensively. He replied that he should talk to Alan about some ground rules, specifically asking if he is comfortable talking about his sexual needs with his nurse.

He realized then that he needed to talk to Alan's home manager about what had happened and agree with Alan his confidentiality issues. Michael was thinking strategically now and creating a tailor-made care plan for this client. He continued to say that he would involve Alan in a learning package where he can learn to be safe, both legally and sexually. Michael cringed as he thought of his spontaneous, albeit well meant, intervention. He realized that he had been on a mission to get Alan away from the public toilets at all cost, but his haste had rendered Alan as disempowered as before.

The tenets of normalization are now widely used to underpin services for people with learning disabilities, but despite their usefulness and sustaining a coherent vision of 'ordinariness' and integration for people using services, an ordinary sexual life continues to elude people. Scandinavian models of normalization (Nirje 1972) rested on the assertion of the rights of people with disabilities, rights that are enshrined in the United Nations Declaration (1971) and which are frequently stated in policies and statements of intent towards people with learning disabilities with regard to sexual issues. Despite this, the recognition of abstract rights has failed to break through the barriers of prejudice and isolation, to create real opportunities for people with learning disabilities to live different kinds of partnerships and family groups, or to enjoy a range of sexual relationships, contacts and activities.

As a practitioner, it is necessary to consider if this is a failure of vision or of implementation. The questions raised relate to whether there is sufficient clarity about what constitutes valued sexual behaviour and relationships for services to have clear and consistent goals. Are there contradictions when these behaviours are engaged in by people with a learning disability? Furthermore, is there an unwillingness or an inability on the part of services (and the individual practitioner) to create opportunities for sexual relationships, to support people in sexual partnerships, and why have services not helped (encouraged) people to live as couples, rather than in group homes? Why has there been no emergence of sexuality 'coaches', relationship finding agencies or marriage brokerage? It has been shown in the implementation of all the other characteristics of social integration that such rigorous strategies can work, so why have they not been adopted to open real sexual options?

Fears and myths about sexuality have long since been projected onto people with learning disabilities. They are framed as asexual or oversexed, innocents or perverts. Historically, service models have been predicated on the need to maintain sexual boundaries between people with learning disabilities and the general public. 'Innocence' models suggest the need to protect people with learning disabilities from predatory members of the public, while 'degenerate' models stressed the need to protect the public from people with learning disabilities. More recently, the documenting of sexual abuse against vulnerable adults has led to boundaries being re-emphasized (Brown and Turk 1992; Turk and Brown 1993).

Meanwhile some people with learning disabilities express their sexual alienation in terms of challenging sexual behaviour, which stigmatizes them as well as abusing others (Turk and Brown 1993). Competence within services to deal with such behaviour is patchy. Serious offending is often overlooked and rationalized as an inevitable concomitant of disability, while minor transgressions are allowed for want of guidance or respect of privacy. Deregulated and smaller services make it less likely that individuals will receive proper services in this area of their lives and lessen the chance that individual staff will build up their expertise in dealing with complex sexual behaviours.

Policies and staff guidelines have been an important starting point, but need now to be translated into individual and service level contracts, so that people's rights are safeguarded and they are not subjected to the whims of individual home owners or managers. This is particularly important for men and women with learning disabilities who wish to have homosexual relationships, who may not be supported in their decisions or assisted in linking into the local gay or lesbian community. Rather than viewing people as living in the community, it may be more useful for practitioners to see their clients as living in or between several communities. Creating networks that provide people with learning disabilities with opportunities to validate their experiences and express themselves more assertively is an essential task. An active support model would involve changes at all levels. In individual work, it would include taking a proactive stance in the face of loneliness or isolation, and being willing to help individuals to meet potential partners or to maintain existing contacts.

Meanwhile, service options need to reflect a greater range of living opportunities than is currently available. The rigidity of housing options for people with learning disabilities means that relationships and gender are not taken into account. Women-only services are not available, nor are services which enable men and women with learning disabilities to live with children, whether their own or other children, who need residential care. Individuals who assert their right to equal treatment in an unequal society inevitably become highly visible, and carry the uncomfortable burden of being a representative of that group. Becoming a champion, while more rewarding than being a token, loads mistakes with awe inspiring significance, which become a liability to those who come after you. Within services, staff need to be willing to engage with parents (Rose and Jones 1993), and to advocate more consistently on behalf of people with learning disabilities to the general public. The aim would not be to challenge the family's own sexual values, but to explore the possibilities of including and supporting individuals with learning disabilities within the same cultural niche and religious traditions.

Practitioners also need to make contact with generic agencies that provide sexuality counselling and support, not only as a way of dealing with a crisis, such as assault or 'coming out', or a way of obtaining services (such as contraception or STD clinics) but as a route to creating networks that acknowledge and support people in their sexual lives. Giving up on sexuality is too high a price to pay; as Pharr (1993: 2) says in the context of challenging homophobia,

> It is a question of wholeness. It is very difficult for one to be denied the life of a sexual being, whether expressed in sex or in physical affection, and to feel complete, whole. For our loving relationships with humans feed the life of the spirit and enable us to overcome our basic isolation and to be interconnected with humankind.

Living an ordinary life is a challenge, but living an ordinary sexual life in the sense of exercising rights over your sexuality is to live a life of defiance. As yet, it is a life that services have done little to support.

◯ Conclusion

The content of this chapter collectively reflects the chapter title; the case studies identify new and different approaches to practice. Practice development can offer innovative solutions to old problems, and the opportunity for community nurses to design and provide alternative services that have a positive health benefit for individuals and the community. The themes highlighted in each case study are important issues for community nurses to consider when embarking upon the journey of developing practice.

Case study 1 demonstrated the importance of networking and communication. Community nurses seeking to influence changes in practice need to recognize and understand the factors that facilitate the communication process, as well as the commonly occurring obstacles. Effective communication is an essential tool for making change, for it serves to both coordinate and control the functioning of individuals and groups and is the means by which shared meaning and understanding is created. Together with establishing supportive networks, communication provides a sound basis for effectively managing the process of developing practice.

Case study 2 identified how professional experience can provide the evidence for practice development. Chapter 2 considered the sources of evidence that community nurses can utilize as a base or a trigger for practice development. Professional experience can be as powerful as any other source of evidence as a stimulus for community nurses to find alternative approaches to nursing practice.

Case study 3 demonstrated the importance of leadership. Leadership is the very process of moving people in some direction; it is the capacity to harness human and other resources to achieve results, and is therefore a central concept in practice development. Leadership will provide the vision, motivation and the support necessary in achieving the task in hand. Implementing successful change is dependent upon good leaders, whose job is to create a vision of what they and others working alongside want to achieve, sell that vision, gain and maintain the involvement and commitment and sense of partnership of others, and support individuals and groups in the pursuit of that objective. Thus building a skill base that allows the leader to become creator, coach, counsellor, facilitator, encourager, builder, partner and nurturer, as the need arises, is crucial.

Finally case study 4 examined the issues of empowerment. It highlighted how community nurses can identify the way in which power is exercised between the nurse and the patient. Empowerment promotes autonomy and helps patients to make informed choices about their care. It provides real opportunities for community nurses to broaden their perspectives, from the often narrow professional viewpoint to the wider horizons of the patient, in discovering how the patient's needs might be most appropriately and effectively met. The case study alerts community nurses to be aware that the professional role and the tradition of 'care' within nursing may be at odds with the whole concept of empowerment, a concept that remains rather imprecise in practice today, its diversity of use adding to its ambiguity.

○ References

Allison, M. (1995) Education and professional development in specialist practice, *British Journal of Nursing*, 4(17): 1005–8.

Angeras, M.H., Brandberg, A., Falk, A. and Seeman, T. (1992) A comparison between sterile saline and tap water for the cleaning of acute traumatic soft tissue wounds, *European Journal of Surgery*, 158(6): 347–50.

Ansell, J.E. (1998) Anticoagulation management as a risk factor for adverse events: grounds for improvement, *Journal of Thrombosis and Thrombolsis*, 5: 13–18.

Association for Continence Advice (1993) *Guidelines for Continence Care.* London: ACA.

Audit Commission (1999a) *First Assessment: A Review of District Nursing Services in England and Wales.* London: Audit Commission.

Audit Commission (1999b) *Listen Up! Effective Community Consultation.* London: Audit Commission.

Bagnall, P. and Dilloway, M. (1997) *In a Different Light: School Nurses and Their Role in Meeting the Needs of School-age Children.* London: Department of Health.

Balfour, M. and Clarke, C.L. (2001) Searching for sustainable change, *Journal of Clinical Nursing*, 10: 44–50.

Balogh, R. (1996) Exploring the links between audit and the research process, *Nurse Researcher*, 3(3): 5–16.

BBC (1998) Health: Care in the Community Failures, *BBC News Online*, 23 November. http://news6.thdo.bbc.co.uk/hi/english/health/newsid_218381.stm

BBC (1999a) UK farming profits halved, *BBC News Online*, 14 October. http://news6.thdo.bbc.co.uk/hi/english/uk/newsid%5F474000/474298.stm

BBC (1999b) Stress and suicide in the country, *BBC News Online*, 13 September. http://news6.thdo.bbc.co.uk/hi/english/special_report/1999/09/99farming_in_crisis/newsid_441000/441895.stm

Beck, U. (1992) *Risk Society: Towards a New Modernity.* London: Sage.

Belbin, M. (1993) *Team Roles at Work.* Oxford: Butterworth-Heinemann.

Benner, P. (1984) *From Novice to Expert: Excellence and Power in Clinical Nursing Practice.* Menlo Park, CA: Addison-Wesley.

Bennis, U. (1990) *Why Can't Leaders Lead?* San Francisco, CA: Jossey-Bass.

Bircumshaw, D. (1990) The utilisation of research findings in clinical practice, *Journal of Advanced Nursing*, 15: 1272–80.

Birkett, M. (1995) Is audit action research? *Physiotherapy*, 81: 190.

Black, S. and Hagel, D. (1996) Developing an integrated nursing team approach, *Health Visitor*, 69(7): 280–3.

Boyd, E.M. and Fales, A.W. (1983) Reflective learning: key to learning from experience, *Journal of Humanistic Psychology*, 23(2): 97–117.

Brett, J.L. (1987) Use of nursing practice research findings, *Nursing Research*, 36(6): 344–9.

British Medical Association (1999) Walk-in centres – not a panacea for the ills of the NHS say GPs, *British Medical Association Press Release*, 13 April.

British Paediatric Association (1993) *Flexible Options for Paediatric Care*, London: BPA.

Brown, H. and Turk, V. (1992) Defining sexual abuse as it affects adults with learning disabilities, *Mental Handicap*, 20(2): 44–5.

Bryans, A. and McIntosh, J. (1996) Decision making in community nursing: an analysis of the stages of decision making as they relate to community nursing practice, *Journal of Advanced Nursing*, 24: 24–30.

Burgess, D. (1996) An evaluation of the ability of senior student nurses to identify ergonomic and other risks to carers arising from moving and handling patients and loads. Unpublished MSc dissertation, University of Northumbria at Newcastle.

Burnard, P. (1989) Developing critical ability in nurse education, *Nurse Education Today*, 9: 271–5.

Bushy, A. (1992) Managing change: strategies for continuing education, *The Journal of Continuing Education in Nursing*, 23: 197–9.

Campbell, C., Wood, R. and Kelly, M. (1999) *Social Capital and Health*. London: Health Education Authority.

Carr, E. (1996) Reflecting on clinical practice: hectoring talk or reality? *Journal of Clinical Nursing*, 5(5): 289–95.

Carson, S. (1999) Organisational change, in S. Hamer and G. Collinson (eds) *Achieving Evidence Based Practice: A Handbook for Practitioners*. Edinburgh: Bailliere Tindall.

Carter, C.E. (1999) The family caring experiences of married women in dementia care, in T. Adams and C.L. Clarke (eds) *Dementia Care: Developing Partnerships in Practice*. London: Bailliere Tindall.

Cauthorne-Lindstrom, C. and Tracy, T. (1992) Organizational change from the 'mom and pop' perspective, *Journal of Nursing Administration*, 22: 61–4.

Chell, E. (1998) Critical incident technique, in G. Symon and C. Cassell (eds) *Qualitative Methods and Analysis in Organisational Research*. London: Sage.

Clarke, C.L. (1997) *Developing Health Care Practice: A Facilitated Seminar Programme*. Newcastle-upon-Tyne: University of Northumbria.

Clarke, C.L. (1999a) Dementia care partnerships: knowledge, ownership and exchange, in T. Adams and C.L. Clarke (eds) *Dementia Care: Developing Partnerships in Practice*. London: Bailliere Tindall.

Clarke, C.L. (1999b) Commentary: a response to Lyons, K.S. and Zarit, S.H. (1999) Formal and informal support: the great divide, *International Journal of Geriatric Psychiatry*, 14: 183–96.

Clarke, C.L. (2000) Risk: constructing care and care environments in dementia, *Health, Risk and Society*, 2(1): 83–93.

Clarke, C.L. and Heyman, B. (1998) Risk management for people with dementia, in B. Heyman (ed.) *Risk, Health and Health Care*. London: Arnold.

Clarke, C.L. and Procter, S. (1999) Practice development: ambiguity in research and practice, *Journal of Advanced Nursing*, 30(4): 975–82.

Clarke, C.L., Procter, S. and Watson, B. (1998) Making changes: a survey to identify mediators in the development of health care practice, *Journal of Clinical Effectiveness in Nursing*, 2: 30–6.

Closs, S.J. and Cheater, F.M. (1999) Evidence for nursing practice: a clarification of the issues, *Journal of Advanced Nursing*, 30(1): 10–17.

Community Practitioners and Health Visitors Association (1996) *Integrated Nursing Teams*, CPHVA Professional Briefing. CPHVA: London.

Community Practitioners and Health Visitors Association (2000) *School Nursing: A National Framework for Practice*. London: CPHVA.

Conroy, M. and Shannon, W. (1995) Clinical guidelines – their implications in general practice, *British Journal of General Practice*, 45: 371–5.

Conway, J. (1994) Reflection, the art and science of nursing and the theory–practice gap, *British Journal of Nursing*, 3(3): 114–18.

Cook, G. (1996) Risk taking in rehabilitative care: professional and legal considerations, *Health Care in Later Life*, 1: 1–15.

Cornwall, A. and Jewkes, R. (1995) What is participatory research? *Social Science and Medicine*, 41: 1667–76.

Coulter, M. (1990) A review of two theories of learning and their application in the practice of nurse education, *Nurse Education Today*, 10: 333–8.

Dahl, R. (1957) The concept of power, *Behavioral Science*, 2: 201–15, in G. Morgan (ed.) (1997) *Images of Organization*. Thousand Oaks, CA: Sage.

Damanpour, F. (1987) The adoption of technological, administrative and ancillary innovations: impact of organizational factors, *Journal of Management*, 13: 675–88.

De Rivera, J. (1976) *Field Theory as Human Science*. New York: Gardner.

Department for Education and Employment (DfEE) (1997) *Excellence in Schools*. London: DfEE.

Department of Health (DoH) (1989) *Working for Patients*, Cmd 555. London: HMSO.

Department of Health (DoH) (1990) *The NHS and Community Care Act*. London: HMSO.

Department of Health (DoH) (1992) *Health of the Nation: A Strategy for Health in England*, Cm 1986. London: HMSO.

Department of Health (DoH) (1996a) *Child Health in the Community: A Guide to Good Practice*. London: DoH.

Department of Health (DoH) (1996b) *The Challenges for Nursing and Midwifery in the 21st Century*, The Heathrow Debate. London: The Stationery Office.

Department of Health (DoH) (1996c) *Promoting Clinical Effectiveness – A Framework for Action In and Through the NHS*. London: The Stationery Office.

Department of Health (DoH) (1997a) *The New NHS: Modern, Dependable*, Cm 3807. London: The Stationery Office.

Department of Health (DoH) (1997b) *Health Action Zones – Invitation to Bid*, EL(97)65. London: DoH.

Department of Health (DoH) (1997c) *Corporate Governance in the NHS: Controls Assurance Statements*, EL(97)55. London: Department of Health.

Department of Health (DoH) (1998a) *Personal Medical Service Pilots – Second Wave*, HSC 1998/176. London: DoH.

Department of Health (DoH) (1998b) *Partnership in Action – New Opportunities for Joint Working between Health and Social Services*. London: DoH.

Department of Health (DoH) (1998c) *Modernising Mental Health Services: Safe, Sound and Supportive*. London: DoH.

Department of Health (DoH) (1998d) *A First Class Service: Quality in the New NHS*. London: Department of Health.

Department of Health (DoH) (1998e) *In the Public Interest: Developing a Strategy for Public Participation in the NHS*. Cambridge: The Bridge Consultancy.

Department of Health (DoH) (1999a) *Saving Lives: Our Healthier Nation*, Cm 4386. London: The Stationery Office.

Department of Health (DoH) (1999b) *Sure Start*, HSC 1999/002. London: DoH.

Department of Health (DoH) (1999c) *Making a Difference: Strengthening the Nursing, Midwifery and Health Visiting Contribution to Health and Healthcare*. London: DoH.

Department of Health (DoH) (1999d) *Facing the Facts: Services for People with Learning Disabilities*. London: DoH.

Department of Health (DoH) (1999e) *National Service Framework for Mental Health*, HSC 1999/223. London: DoH.

Department of Health (DoH) (1999f) *Reform of the Mental Health Act 1983: Proposals for Consultation*, Cm 4480. London: The Stationery Office.

Department of Health (DoH) (2000a) *The NHS Plan: A Plan for Investment. A Plan for Reform*, Cm 4818–1. London: HMSO.

Department of Health (DoH) (2000b) *Go-Ahead for Plans to Allow Nurses to Prescribe More Medicines*, DoH Press Release 2000/0146. London: DoH.

Department of Health (DoH) (2000c) *Shaping the Future NHS: Long Term Planning for Hospitals and Related Services*, The National Beds Inquiry. London: DoH.

Department of Health and Social Security (DHSS) (1983) *NHS Management Enquiry*, The Griffiths Report. London: DHSS.

Department of Health and Social Services (DHSS) (1999) *Working Together: A Focus for Modern Health and Social Services Well-being*. Belfast: DHSS Northern Ireland.

Dickson, R. (1996a) Dissemination and implementation: the wider picture, *Nurse Researcher*, 4(1): 5–14.

Dickson, R. (1996b) Developing guidelines for clinical practice, *Nurse Researcher*, 4(2): 5–14.

Dirschel, K.M. (1996) Managing conflict, in B.L. Marquis and C.J. Huston (eds) *Leadership Roles and Management Functions in Nursing*, 2nd edn. Philadelphia, PA: Lippincott-Raven.

Droogan, J. and Song, F. (1996) The process and importance of systematic reviews, *Nurse Researcher*, 4(1): 15–26.

Drucker, P. (1996) Foreword, in F. Hessembein, M. Goldsmith and R. Beckhard (eds) *The Leader of the Future*. San Francisco, CA: Jossey-Bass.

Drury, M., Greenfield, S., Stillwell, B. and Hull, F.M. (1988) A nurse practitioner in general practice: patient perceptions and expectations, *Journal of the Royal College of General Practitioners*, 38(316): 503–5.

Edmonds, M., May, T., Hernden, I. and Hough, M. (1998) *Arrest Referral: Emerging Lessons from Research*. London: Home Office.

Edwards, K. (1995) What are nurses' views on expanding practice? *Nursing Standard*, 9(41): 38–40.

English National Board (ENB) (1998) *Occupational Health Nursing: Contributing to Healthier Workplaces*. London: English National Board for Nursing Midwifery and Health Visiting.

Eraut, M. (1994) *Developing Professional Knowledge and Competence*. The Falmer Press: London.

Ferguson, K.E. and Jinks, A.M. (1994) Integrating what is taught with what is practiced in the nursing curriculum: a multidimensional model, *Journal of Advanced Nursing*, 20: 687–95.

Fisher, R., Ury, W. and Patton, B. (1992) *Getting to Yes: Negotiating an Agreement Without Giving In*, 2nd edn. London: Random House Business Books.

Fitzgerald, M. (1994) Theories of reflection for learning, in A. Palmer, S. Burns and C. Bulman (eds) *Reflective Practice in Nursing: The Growth of the Professional Programme*. Oxford: Blackwell Science.

Flanagan, M. (1997) Guidelines and protocols in clinical decision making, *Journal of Wound Care*, 6(5): 207.

Freire, P. (1972) *Pedagogy of the Oppressed*. London: Penguin.

Garbett, R. (1996) The growth of nurse led care, *Nursing Times*, 92(1): 29.

Garland, G. and Corefield, F. (1999) Audit, in S. Hamer and G. Collinson (eds) *Achieving Evidence Based Practice*. Edinburgh: Bailliere Tindall.

Gerrish, K. and Ferguson, A. (2000) Nursing development units: factors influencing their progress, *British Journal of Nursing*, 9(10): 626–30.

Gossop, M., Marsden, J. and Stewart, D. (1998) *The National Treatment Outcome Research Study at One Year*. London: Department of Health.

Greenwood, J. (1984) Nursing research: a position paper, *Journal of Advanced Nursing*, 9(1): 77–82.

Griffiths, P. (1999) The challenge of implementing evidence-based healthcare, *British Journal of Community Nursing*, 4(3): 142–7.

Haffer, A. (1986) Facilitating change: choosing the appropriate strategy, *Journal of Nursing Administration*, 16: 18–22.

Hamer, S. and Collinson, G. (eds) (2000) *Achieving Evidence-Based Practice. A Handbook for Practitioners*. London: Bailliere Tindall.

Harden, J. (1996) Enlightenment, empowerment and emancipation: the case for critical pedagogy in nurse education, *Nurse Education Today*, 16(1), 32–7.

Hargreaves, J. (1997) Using patients: exploring the ethical dimension of reflective practice in nurse education, *Journal of Advanced Nursing*, 25(2): 223–8.

Hart, E. and Bond, M. (1995) *Action Research for Health and Social Care: A Guide to Practice*. Buckingham: Open University Press.

Hayes, M.V. (1992) On the epistemology of risk: language, logic and social science, *Social Science and Medicine*, 35(4): 401–6.

Health and Safety Executive (HSE) (1998) *Developing an Occupational Health Strategy for Great Britain*. London: HSE.

Hesketh, J. (1999) Making a difference – the new nursing strategy, *The Queen's Nursing Institute Newsletter*, 9(4): 1.

Heyman, B. (1998) *Risk, Health and Health care*. London: Arnold.

Heyman, B. and Henriksen, M. (2000) *Age, Risk and Pregnancy.* London: Macmillan.

Home Office (1998a) *Supporting Families: A Consultation Document.* London: Home Office.

Home Office (1998b) *Tackling Drugs to Build a Better Britain,* Cm 3945. London: HMSO.

Home Office (1999) *Supporting Families: Summary of Responses to the Consultation Document.* London: Home Office.

Hopkins, C., Benjamin, C. and Carter, A. (1997) *Regeneration: Some Legal and Practical Issues.* http://www.lawgram.com/regen.html

Hunt, J. (1984) Why don't we use these findings? *Nursing Mirror,* 158: 29.

Hurst, K. (1985) Traditional versus progressive nurse education: a review of the literature, *Nurse Education Today,* 5: 30–6.

James, C.R. and Clarke, B.A. (1994) Reflective practice in nursing: issues and implications for nurse education, *Nurse Education Today,* 14: 82–90.

Johnson, B. (1999) Ethical issues in risk communication: continuing the discussion, *Risk Analysis,* 19(3): 335–48.

Johnson, M. (1994) Conflict and nursing professionalisation, in J. McCloskey and H.K. Grace (eds) *Current Issues in Nursing,* 4th edn. St Louis, MO: C.V. Mosby.

Joyce, L. (1999) Development of practice, in S. Hamer and G. Collinson (eds) *Achieving Evidence Based Practice: A Handbook for Practitioners.* Edinburgh: Bailliere Tindall.

Kendall, S. (1997) What do we mean by evidence? implications for primary health care nursing, *Journal of Interprofessional Care,* 11(1): 23–34.

Kimberly, J.R. and Evanisko, M.J. (1981) Organizational innovation: the influence of individual, organisational and contextual factors on hospital adoption of technological and administrative innovations, *Academy of Management Journal,* 24: 689–713.

King, N. (1989) Innovation in elderly care organisations: process and attitudes. Unpublished PhD thesis: University of Sheffield.

King, N. and Anderson, N. (1995) *Innovation and Change in Organisations.* London: Routledge.

Kitzinger, J. (1995) Introducing focus groups, *British Medical Journal,* 311: 299–301.

Kramer, M. (1990) The magnet hospitals: excellence revisited, *Journal of Nursing Administration,* 20(9): 35–44.

Krueger, R.A. (1988) *Focus Groups: A Practical Guide for Applied Research.* Newbury Park, CA: Sage.

Lancaster, J. (1999) *Nursing issues in leading and managing change.* St Louis, MO: Mosby.

Lancaster, J. and Lancaster, W. (1983) *Concepts of Advanced Nursing Practice: The Nurse as a Change Agent.* New York: Mosby.

Langford, T. (1981) *Managing and Being Managed.* Englewood Cliffs, NJ: Prentice Hall.

Lathlean, J. (1997) *Lecturer Practitioners in Action.* Oxford: Butterworth-Heinemann.

Lewin, K. (1951) *Field Theory in Social Sciences.* New York: Harper Row.

Lewin, K. (1958) Group decision and social change, in E.E. Maccoby, T.M. Newcomb and E.L. Hartley (eds) *Readings in Social Psychology,* 3rd edn. New York: Holt.

Lippitt, G.L. (1973) *Visualizing Change: Model Building and the Change Process*. Fairfax: NTL Learning Resources Corporation.

Logue, R. (1996) Is nursing research detrimental to nursing education and practice? *Nurse Researcher*, 4(1): 63–9.

Lyons, K.S. and Zarit, S.H. (1999) Formal and informal support: the great divide, *International Journal of Geriatric Psychiatry*, 14: 183–96.

McCormack, B., Manley, K., Kitson, A., Titchen, A. and Harvey, G. (1999) Towards practice development: a vision in reality or a reality without vision? *Journal of Nursing Management*, 7: 255–64.

Mackenzie, A. and Ross, F. (1997) Shifting the balance: nursing in primary care, *British Journal of Community Health Nursing*, 2(3): 139–42.

Mackintosh, C. (1998) Reflection: a flawed strategy for the nursing profession, *Nurse Education Today*, 18(7): 553–7.

Manion, J. (1993) Chaos or transformation, *Journal of Nursing Administration*, 23(5): 41–8.

Marquis, B.L. and Huston, C.J. (1996) *Leadership Roles and Management Functions in Nursing*. Philadelphia, PA: Lippincott-Raven.

Mason, D.J., Costello-Nickitas, D.M., Scanlon, J.M. and Magnuson, B.A. (1991) Empowering nurses for politically astute change in the workplace, *The Journal of Continuing Education in Nursing*, 22: 5–10.

Meyer, J. and Batehup, L. (1997) Action research in health-care practice: nature, present concerns and future possibilities, *Nursing Times Research*, 2: 175–84.

Mezirow, J. (1981) A critical theory of adult learning and education, *Adult Education*, 32(1): 3–24.

Mintzberg, H. (1979) *The Structure of Organizations*. Englewood Cliffs, NJ: Prentice Hall.

Morgan, G. (1997) *Images of Organization*. Thousand Oaks, CA: Sage Publications.

Morgan, M.G. and Lave, L. (1990) Ethical considerations in risk communication practice and research, *Risk Analysis*, 10: 355–8.

Moscovici, S. (1976) *Social Influence and Social Change*. London: Academic Press.

Mugford, M., Banfield, P. and O'Hanlon, M. (1991) Effects of feedback of information on clinical practice: a review, *British Medical Journal*, 303: 398–402.

Muir Gray, J.A. (1997) *Evidence Based Healthcare: How to Make Health Policy and Management Decisions*. Edinburgh: Churchill Livingstone.

Mulhall, A. (1995) Nursing research: what difference does it make? *Journal of Advanced Nursing*, 21: 576–83.

National Assembly for Wales (1999) *Realising Potential*. Cardiff: National Assembly for Wales.

Newburn, T. and Elliott, J. (1998) *Police Anti-Drug Strategies*, Crime detection and prevention series, Paper 89, Police Research Group. London: Home Office.

NHS Centre for Reviews and Dissemination (1999) Treating head lice and scabies, *Effectiveness Matters*, 4(1): 1–6.

NHS Executive (1996a) *NHS Annual Report 1995/96*. London: NHSE.

NHS Executive (1996b) *Clinical Audit in the NHS: Using Clinical Audit in the NHS, A Position Statement*. Leeds: NHSE.

NHS Executive (1997) *R & D in Primary Care, National Working Group Report*. Leeds: NHSE.

NHS Management Executive (1991) *Junior Doctors: The New Deal.* London: NHSME.

NHS Management Executive (1993) *Risk Management in the NHS.* Leeds: NHSME.

Nirje, B. (1972) The right to self determination, in W. Wolfensberger (ed.) *The Principle of Normalization in Human Services.* Toronto: National Institute of Mental Retardation.

Norman, A. (1980) *Rights and Risk,* 2nd edn. London: Centre for Policy on Ageing.

Northern Ireland Office (1997) *Well into 2000.* Belfast: Department of Health and Social Services.

Northern Ireland Office (1998) *Fit for the Future.* Belfast: Department of Health and Social Services.

Office for National Statistics (1999) *Social Trends 29.* London: The Stationery Office.

Office for National Statistics (2000) *Annual Abstract of Statistics, 2000 edition.* London: The Stationery Office.

OXCHECK Study Group (1995) Effectiveness of health checks conducted by nurses in primary care: final results of the OXCHECK study, *British Medical Journal,* 310: 1099–104.

Oxford University Press (1992) Oxford English Dictionary. Oxford: Oxford University Press.

Palmer, R.H., Louis, T.A., Hsu, L.N. *et al.* (1995) A randomised controlled trial of quality assurance in sixteen ambulatory care practices, *Medical Care,* 23(1): 751–70.

Pearson, A. (1983) *The Clinical Nursing Unit.* London: Heinemann.

Pearson, P., Kelly, A., Connolly, M., Daly, M. and O'Gorman, F. (1995) Nurse practitioners, *Health Visitor,* 68(4): 157–60.

Peters, T.J. and Waterman, R.H. (1982) *In Search of Excellence: Lessions from America's Best Run Companies.* London: Harper Row.

Pharr, S. (1993) Homophobia: a weapon of sexism, *Siecus Report,* 21(3): 1–4.

Phillips, C., Palfrey, C. and Thomas, P. (1994) *Evaluating Health and Social Care.* London: Macmillan.

Poyner, B. and Warne, C. (1986) *Violence to staff: A Basis for Assessment and Intervention.* London: HMSO.

Primary Health Care Development (1999) *Simple Guide to PMS Pilots.* London: PHD.

Procter, S. (1999) Practice development. Paper presented to the Royal College of Nursing Action Research Conference, Leeds, 23 June.

Quinn, F. (1995) *The Principles and Practice of Nurse Education.* Cheltenham: Stanley Thornes.

Rafferty, A.M., Allcock, N. and Lathlean, J. (1996) The theory/practice gap: taking issue with the issue, *Journal of Advanced Nursing,* 23(4): 685–91.

Ranade, W. (1997) *A Future for the NHS: Health Care for the Millennium.* London: Longman.

Reed, J. and Procter, S. (1995) Practitioner research in context, in J. Reed and S. Procter (eds) *Practitioner Research in Health Care: The Inside Story.* London: Chapman & Hall.

Reilly, R. and Perrin, C. (1999) Preparing the nursing profession: educating to lead or training to be manageable? *The Australian Electronic Journal of Nursing Education,* 4(2). http://www.scu.edu.au/schools/nhcp/aejne/vol4-2/reillyvol4_2.htm

Riyat, M.S. and Quinton, D.N. (1997) Tap water as a wound cleansing agent in accident and emergency, *Journal of Accident and Emergency Medicine*, 14(3): 165–6.

Rogers, A. (1996) *Teaching Adults*. Buckingham: Open University Press.

Rogers, C. and Freiberg, H. (1994) *Freedom to Learn*. Oxford: Macmillan International.

Rogers, E. and Shoemaker, F. (1971) *Communication of Innovation: A Cross Cultural Approach*. New York: The Free Press.

Rogers, E.M. (1995) *Diffusion of Innovations*, 4th edn. New York: Free Press.

Rolfe, G. (1996) Going to extremes: action research, grounded practice and the theory–practice gap in nursing, *Journal of Advanced Nursing*, 24(6): 1315–20.

Rose, J. and Jones, C. (1993) Working with parents, in A. Craft (ed.) *Practice Issues in Sexuality and Intellectual Disability*. London: Routlege.

Ross, F. and Meerabeau, L. (1997) Editorial: research and professional practice, *Journal of Interprofessional Care*, 11: 5.

Rossi, K. and Heikkinen, M. (1990) A view of occupational health nursing practice: current trends and future prospects, in J.M. Radford (ed.) *Recent Advances in Nursing: Occupational Health Nursing*. Edinburgh: Churchill Livingstone.

Royal College of Nursing (1995) *Clinical Guidelines: What You Need to Know*. London: RCN.

Royal College of Nursing (1996) *Buying Paediatric Community Nursing: A Guide for Purchasers and Commissioners of Health Care*. London: RCN.

Royal College of Physicians (1995) *Incontinence: Causes, Management and Provision of Services*. London: Royal College of Physicians.

The Royal Society (1992) *Risk: Analysis, Perception and Management*, Report of a Royal Society Study Group. London: The Royal Society.

Ryan, T. (1993) Therapeutic risk taking in mental health nursing, *Nursing Standard*, 7: 29–31.

Sackett, D.L., Richardson, W.S., Rosenberg, W. and Hayes, R.B. (1997) *Evidence Based Medicine: How to Practice and Teach EBM*. Edinburgh: Churchill Livingstone.

Salvage, J. and Smith, R. (2000) Doctors and nurses: doing it differently, *British Medical Journal*, 320, 1019–20.

Samuels, A. (1993) The legal liability of the nurse – the lawyer's view, *Medicine, Science and the Law*, 33(4): 305–9.

Scholefield, H.A., Viney, C. and Evans, J. (1997) Expanding practice and obtaining consent, *Professional Nurse*, 13(1): 12–16.

Schön, D.A. (1988) From technical rationality to reflection in action, in J. Cambridge (ed.) *Professional Judgement: A Reader in Clinical Decision Making*. Cambridge: Cambridge University Press.

Schön, D.A. (1991) *The Reflective Practitioner*. San Francisco, CA: Jossey-Bass.

Scottish Office (1997) *Designed to Care: Renewing the NHS in Scotland*, Cm 3811. London: The Stationery Office.

Scottish Office (1999) *Working Together for a Healthier Scotland*, Cm 3854. London: The Stationery Office.

Silverman, J., Kurtz, S. and Draper J. (1998) *Skills for Communicating with Patients*. Oxford: Radcliffe Medical Press.

Sines, D. (1995) Community learning disabilities nursing, in D. Sines (ed.) *Community Health Care Nursing*. London: Blackwell.

Social Exclusion Unit (1998) *Bringing Britain Together: A National Strategy for Neighbourhood Renewal*, Cmd 4045. London: The Stationery Office.

Social Exclusion Unit (1999) *Teenage Pregnancy*, Cm 4342. London: The Stationery Office.

Steiner, A. and Vaughan, B. (1996) *Intermediate Care: A Conceptual Framework and Review of the Literature*. London: The King's Fund.

Street, A. (1991) *From Image to Action – Reflection in Nursing Practice*. Geelong: Deakin University.

Swage, T. (2000) *Clinical Governance in Health Care Practice*. Oxford: Butterworth-Heinemann.

Taylor, B. (2000) *Reflective Practice: A Guide for Nurses and Midwives*. Buckingham: Open University Press.

Tingle, J. (1995) Clinical protocols and the law, *Nursing Times*, 91(29): 27–8.

Tingle, J. (1998) Developing clinical guidelines: present and future legal aspects, *British Journal of Nursing*, 7(11): 672–4.

Turk, V. and Brown, H. (1993) The sexual abuse of adults with learning disabilities: results of a two year incidence survey, *Mental Handicap Research*, 6(3): 3–24.

UKCC (1992a) *The Scope of Professional Practice*. London: UKCC.

UKCC (1992b) *Code of Professional Conduct for Nurses, Midwives and Health Visitors*. London: UKCC.

UKCC (1994) *The Future of Professional Practice – The Council's Standards for Education and Practice Following Registration: Programmes of Education Leading to the Qualification of Specialist Practitioner*. London: UKCC.

UKCC (2000) *The Scope of Professional Practice – A Study of its Implementation*. London: United Kingdom Central Council for Nursing, Midwifery and Health Visiting.

Ungerson, C. (1987) *Policy is Personal – Sex, Gender and Informal Care*. London: Tavistock.

United Nations (1971) *Declaration of General and Special Rights of the Mentally Handicapped*. New York: United Nations Department of Social Affairs.

Unsworth, J. (2000) Practice development: a concept analysis, *Journal of Nursing Management*, 8(6): 317–26.

Unsworth, J., Hardy, L., Binks, E. and Patterson, T. (2000) District nursing involvement in intermediate care, *Journal of Community Nursing*, 14: 21–5.

US Department of Health and Human Services (1992) *Urinary Incontinence in Adults: Clinical Practice Guidelines*. Rockville, MD: Agency for Health Care Policy and Research Public Health Service.

Vincent, C. (1995) *Clinical Risk Management*. London: BMJ Publishing Group.

von Degenberg, K. (1996) Clinical guidelines: improving practice at local level, *Nursing Standard*, 10(19): 37–9.

Walker, L.O. and Avant, K.C. (1995) *Strategies for Theory Construction in Nursing*, 3rd edn. Norwalk, CT: Appleton Lange.

Wallis, S. (1998) Changing practice through action research, *Nurse Researcher*, 6(2): 5–15.

Walshe, K. and Dineen, M. (1998) *Clinical Risk Management: Making a Difference*. Birmingham: The NHS Confederation.

Watson, B. and Heyman, B. (1998) Risk and coping with diabetes, in B. Heyman (ed.) *Risk, Health and Health Care*. London: Arnold.

Welsh Office (1998a) *NHS Wales: Putting Patients First*, Cm 3841. London: The Stationery Office.

Welsh Office (1998b) *Better Health: Better Wales*, Cm 3922. London: The Stationery Office.

West, M. (1999) Communication and teamworking in healthcare, *NT Research*, 4: 8–14.

West, M.A. and Anderson, N.R. (1992) Innovation, cultural values and the management of change in British hospitals, *Work and Stress*, 6: 293–310.

West, M.A. and Farr, J.L. (1990) *Innovation and Creativity at Work*. Chichester: John Wiley and Sons.

West, M.A. and Wallace, M. (1991) Innovation in health care teams, *European Journal of Social Psychology*, 21: 303–15.

While, A.E. (1991) An evaluation of a paediatric home care scheme, *Journal of Advanced Nursing*, 16: 1413–21.

Willis, J. (1998) Last among equals, *Nursing Times*, 94: 16–17.

Wilson, J. (1995) Clinical risk modification, *British Journal of Nursing*, 4(11): 667.

Wilson, J. and Tingle, J. (1997) Clinical risk modification, *British Journal of Nursing*, 6(18): 1068–9.

Wilson, J. and Tingle, J. (1999) *Clinical Risk Modification: A Route to Clinical Governance?* Oxford: Butterworth-Heinneman.

Wood, N., Farrow, S. and Elliot, B. (1994) A review of primary health care organisation, *Journal of Community Nursing*, 3: 243–250.

Woolf, S. (1990) Practice guidelines: a new reality in medicine: 1 recent developments, *Archives of International Medicine*, 150: 1811–18.

Wright, S. (1987) Defining the nursing development unit, *Nursing Standard*, 4(7): 29–31.

Young, L. (2000) A radical change in primary care, *Primary Health Care*, 10: 18–19.

Zaleznik, A. (1992) Managers and leaders: are they different? *Harvard Business Review*, 70(2): 126–35.

Index

COMMUNITY CARE FOR NURSES AND THE CARING PROFESSIONS

Nigel Malin, Jill Manthorpe, David Race and Stephen Wilmot

This textbook provides a concise introduction to policy and practice issues in community care. It has been written for nurses and other health professionals in training, particularly those wishing to specialize in community care. It explains the concepts behind community care policy and demonstrates their relevance to work in healthcare settings.

In a clear, accessible way, the authors draw together a wide range of material on the changing nature of community care, assess current research evidence and examine the central issues relating to everyday practice. Each chapter has a similar structure, with an introductory and concluding section making it ideal for use as a teaching text. At the end of each chapter there are suggestions for further reading and follow-up work. Students will also find key points and concepts listed throughout the text which are explained in a helpful glossary at the end of the book.

Contents

224pp   0 335 19670 5 (Paperback)   0 335 19671 3 (Hardback)

REFLECTIVE PRACTICE
A GUIDE FOR NURSES AND MIDWIVES

Beverley J. Taylor

Reflection helps us understand the impact of our actions and improve our professional skills. This practical guide shows nurses and midwives how to develop a reflective approach to their work and how to sustain reflective practice throughout their professional lives.

Bev Taylor introduces three main types of reflection: technical, practical and emancipatory, showing readers how these can be used in different aspects of clinical work. She acknowledges the issues faced by practitioners in bureaucratic work settings with time constraints and regulated routines, and shows how reflection can help professionals deal with the complexity of their working lives. Readers are given a 'kitbag' of strategies they can use to get started.

With great warmth Bev Taylor describes how developing a reflective practice is part of learning how to value yourself as a nurse or midwife, and as a person. Throughout the book she provides real examples of reflective writing from nurses and midwives, and shows how these professionals have been able to improve their skills as a result of being alert to their practice.

A practical and insightful guide, richly illuminated with stories from everyday practice, to enable the practitioner to become an effective reflective practitioner. The power of Bev Taylor's approach is to view reflection as a way of life and not just as a technique.
Christopher Johns, Reader in Advanced Nursing Practice,
University of Luton, UK

Bev Taylor's latest work weaves a tapestry for a reflective frame as foundational to our humanity, restoring and integrating the personal with our professional life, work and experiences . . . It is a hopeful framework and a healing gift to all practising nurses and midwives.
Jean Watson, Distinguished Professor of Nursing,
University of Colorado, USA

Contents
The nature of reflection – The nature of nursing and midwifery – Getting ready to reflect – Practitioners' reflections on their personal histories – The value of reflection – Types of reflection – Technical reflection – Practical reflection – Emancipatory reflection – Experiences and reflections – Maintaining reflective practice – References – Index.

272pp   0 335 20689 1 (Paperback)   0 335 20690 5 (Hardback)